Paths to Healthy Aging

A Workbook by Mehrdad Ayati, M.D.
and Arezou Azarani, Ph.D.

Edited by Philip L. Hubbard, Ph.D.

DEDICATION

To our parents, our grandparents and our patients with much love and gratitude.

Table of Contents

Acknowledgement

We would like to thank Jonathan Ray Mendoza for his participation in the exercise pictures.

Disclaimer

The information in this book, true and complete to the best of our knowledge, is intended as an informative guide only. The information in this book is offered with no guarantees on the part of the authors and the authors disclaim all liability in connection with the use of this book. This book is not intended as a substitute for the medical advice of your own physician(s) nor is it intended to replace, conflict with or countermand the advice of your physician(s). The reader should regularly consult a physician in matters relating to his or her health and particularly with respect to any symptoms that may require diagnosis or medical attention. The ultimate decision concerning your care should be made between you and your physician(s). We strongly recommend you follow his or her advice. The names and identifying details of people associated with events described in this book have been changed and any similarity to actual persons is coincidental.

Illustrations

All illustrations and pictures, unless otherwise noted, were purchased from ©Dollar Photo Club (http://www.dollarphotoclub.com/) and are included in this book with permission from Dollar Photo Club. Dollar Photo Club illustrations/picture ID numbers: 20032937, 64921143, 61789687, 56164030, 65486724, 54319396, 60373779, 29519896, 64882203, 60684980, 7305871, 47162666, 65959385, 63277078, 47220216, 61157871, 54705235, 4709589, 39627054, 30233426, 2775908, 64122437, 60287307, 64456642, 58595136, 51287319, 38024040, 61978337, 32957522, 58663120, 66105177, 66105163.

Introduction

I am Mehrdad Ayati, MD, and I will be speaking with you through the pages of this workbook. I was born and raised in Iran until my early thirties, the youngest child in the family. My father, an ophthalmologist, still practices in his early eighties, and my mother (in her seventies), who recently retired to pursue other interests, was a midwife. While my mom got her degree in England, my dad did his education in France. They are both great teachers and mentors, highly respected in their own fields, and have helped thousands of patients throughout their careers. As such they were my role models, and from early on I had decided to follow in their footsteps. My older sister became an OB/GYN and married an orthopedic surgeon. My older brother was the only black sheep in the family—he thought there was something wrong with all of us and became an engineer. He believed that only people with personality disorders wanted to become doctors, and joked to us that most doctors were highly egoistic, utterly snobbish and unapproachable. So of course he ended up marrying a doctor!

After I finished my medical education and started practicing, I thought that similarly to my mom and dad I wanted to pursue further training abroad. There was so much to learn, and I had reached a plateau in my domain. The United States was the obvious choice since all of my precious medical books were written in the States by highly respected professors and dedicated doctors. So on a nice spring day, I declared to my family members that I was leaving my home to move to California. I will not trouble you with all the steps I had to take and all the hurdles I had to overcome to get to California and will leave that for another book. I will only tell you that half of my hair turned white in the process.

When I finally arrived in California I discovered that I had to pass numerous tests and re-do my residency. And then the rest of my hair turned white! When it came down to choosing a residency program the possibilities were endless, and I was like a kid in a candy shop. First, I thought about becoming a GI (gastrointestinal) specialist, and then there were sports medicine, hospitalist, ER medicine, pediatrics, etc. After a period of intense thinking and sleepless nights I finally decided to go to the University of California, Davis and pursue a residency program in family medicine. This specialty allowed me to get exposed to most of the medical subspecialties and to practice on people of all ages. More importantly, it provided me with the range of experience I needed to determine what sub-specialty to pursue.

During the time I did my residency I became highly interested in geriatrics, and at the end, I decided to pursue a fellowship in geriatrics at Stanford University. I remember that during the interview phase I was asked why I chose this subspecialty. There were many reasons why I set my mind on becoming a geriatrician, and I will briefly mention a few here.

Respect and fascination. In my culture the elderly hold a very special status in the society. They are considered very sage, are highly respected and have a central position in the family and their community. Because of the years of experience they have acquired, their words carry a lot of substance and their advice and decisions are highly sought and utterly valued. Understandably, everyone dreams of holding such a prominent status from early in life. Gray hair is considered an asset in our culture, and the day you get your first gray hair you don't dye it. You brag about it.

In Middle Eastern as well as many Asian societies, each family gets its direction and guidance from the eldest person in the household. It is thus an honor to take care of the elderly, listen to their riveting stories, learn from their invaluable experiences and skills, cherish their collected wisdom and follow their path. As such, most families have never heard of senior care facilities or assisted living.

Personal rewards and gratification. We recently had a baby, and it was fascinating how excited our family members, friends, colleagues and mostly my patients became. Everyone pitched in to help. Anyone who has had a baby knows how much hard work and dedication goes into the process. However, nobody minds the constant cries, staying up all night to attend to the baby's needs, changing diapers and getting spit, pee and poop on themselves. We actually enjoy it and find it very enriching! I have heard from everyone that taking care of babies brings us back to our youth and gives us a clean slate or canvas to fill anew taking into account all the wisdom we have acquired along the way.

So babies are great, but as people grow older they also need more attention, care, support, companionship, and love. I enjoy taking care of the elderly and am a big advocate of their physical and mental health. My research continuously focuses on finding practical yet innovative ways of addressing their wellbeing and needs. And I find this relationship to be a two-way symbiosis in that the more I try to help them through my research, the more I enrich my own life. Helping them allows me to fill my life canvas with bright and solid colors via their lifetime experiences.

Duty and appreciation. Our mothers and fathers endured so much to raise us, put us through school, give us roots, and support us through every hardship along the way. They gave us their unlimited love, devotion and attention. They worked hard for decades, paid taxes, and gave our society their best years and youth. In their golden ages the clock turns, and now they need our support, devotion, love and strength.

I believe that our society is not treating our elderly as it should. It is true that we live in a capitalist country. And there is nothing wrong with generating profits and wealth; however, this should not happen on the backs of our elderly. Not everything should be evaluated on a monetary basis. For instance, our elderly should not be forced out of the work force and replaced by cheaper and inexperienced labor. They should not be institutionalized and set aside by the society they built and the children they raised. They should not be taken advantage of, cheated or mistreated in any form or fashion. We owe them our respect, our time, and our gratitude.

Since becoming a geriatrician I have had the privilege to see and treat thousands of patients and interact with their family members. I have heard their fascinating stories, commiserated with their aches and pains, and tried my best to offer them relief, cure when possible, and support. The most interesting observation I have had is that patients primarily want someone to truly listen to them. They want to form a connection with their physicians since it brings along a great deal of trust and faith. Therefore, before they rely on their physician's medical judgment, they want to be assured of his or her personality and integrity. They appreciate kindness, humility and honesty. They want someone who truly cares about them, is attentive to their concerns, follows up with them, and coordinates their care efficiently and seamlessly.

The next thing that is of most interest to patients is valid, up-to-date information on how to prevent, treat or live with diseases. They want to grasp complex medical issues in a comprehensible format. We live during an era where massive amounts of information are available to us at our finger tips. However, the validity of much of this information is highly questionable. Are these theories marketing-oriented, myths, backed by solid evidence or knowledge based? I have often heard complaints on this subject from my patients. They are confused by all the contradictory claims, each professing to be reasonable and authoritative.

Therefore, I set this as a goal for myself. Through attending conferences, reviewing the old to the most recent literature and publications, consulting with other physicians, nurse practitioners, and physical therapists, and conducting research through collaborations with scientists in this field worldwide, I have gained valuable knowledge and experience. I have decided to put that knowledge and experience at the disposal of my patients and other interested readers in the format of a workbook.

This workbook is about creating a "lifestyle" to lead readers toward the path of a healthy and happy aging process. This methodology is not composed of just one element but a combination of factors, which together create a colorful journey. To follow this concept all you need is you and a mind free of everything it has been programmed with thus far via the media on the subject. Let me explain. You have probably read many books and articles, perhaps attended some lectures, and almost certainly listened to experts, friends, colleagues and family members on the topic of aging. And they have combined to confuse you deeply about the right plan to follow in order to stay as healthy as possible and live a long and happy life. They have told you to follow drastic diets, consume over-the-counter supplements, exercise excessively, memorize the phone book to keep dementia at bay, and work as long as possible to save enough money to pay for your health care cost and assisted living or senior care facilities. None of these factors have really helped the public since about 80 percent of seniors have at least one chronic health condition, others have or are at a high risk of getting cancer and all too many are living unhappy lives!

As I mentioned, there is a lot of information out there and most of it is very confusing for my patients and their caregivers. Those recommendations for healthy and happy living are hard and often impossible to follow. In my practice I am faced with many disappointed patients who are exhausted from following these unsuccessful steps. I am inundated with their frustrated comments and questions. My goal here is to clarify a few of these misconceptions and simplify the journey. Based on my experience of what has worked best for my patients to achieve meaningful, joyful and healthy lives, I have put together this simple workbook. I have omitted long explanations and complex medical terms to keep things straightforward. I know your time is precious and will be better spent on additional exciting endeavors.

This workbook contains only a few chapters. At the beginning of each there is a list of questions. Take your time to read them carefully, think about your answers and write them down. The answers will help you when you read the chapter and also when you see your geriatrician. There are no right or wrong answers. Do not stress out if your answers are different from my recommendations. If something has truly been working out for you then you do not need to change it. You can also discuss your concerns with your geriatrician during your next visit and get his or her opinion.

If you decide you need to change something to see a better health outcome, start slowly and take baby steps. Let me give you an example. When patients come to my clinic and need to lose weight I don't want them to lose 50 pounds in two months. I want them to lose one pound every month, if possible. If they lose the weight slowly their bodies don't go into shock and there is a much stronger chance that they will lose the weight and keep it off for years to come. Consequently, the stress will be minimal on their body and mind. Therefore, seek the least stressful and most enjoyable path to achieve the desired outcome.

In the chapters that follow, we will discuss nutrition, mental health, physical health, medications and how to go about choosing the right geriatrician. While reading this book, keep a few points in mind. When it comes to nutrition and the recipe for a healthy balanced diet, moderation is the key. When it comes to mental health, stimulation and exhilaration are the goals. Physical health is achieved not by strenuous exercising but by persistent and yet enjoyable workouts. Before reaching out for any prescription or over-the-counter medication, supplements, and herbal remedies, stop and consult with your physician no matter how much you may have heard about their benefits in the media. Choose a doctor that you can trust, easily engage with and build a long-term relationship with.

Above all, remember that you only have one precious life to live. During each step of the way, think about your actions. If they lead to stress, depression, anxiety and unhappiness, don't go any further until you figure out how to turn the journey into a path of excitement, happiness, jubilation and above all love. You are the only one in charge. Even genes (your genetic makeup) cannot enforce their agenda on your will. Many individuals with severe genetic diseases, people exposed to horrific environmental factors, and those faced with tragic events have lived jovial lives.

A few years back I had the most interesting patient. She was close to ninety years old. She was a precious, proud and energetic retired officer from the Air Force and was in a retirement facility catering to retired veterans. Needless to say, she was the only woman among the many retired Army, Navy and Air Force veterans. She had this unique routine every day, which included rising very early in the morning, swimming for an hour, getting her hair (and sometimes nails) done, putting on her makeup, having breakfast, playing croquet, having lunch, taking a nap in the early afternoon, playing cards followed by having an afternoon tea, going over her mail and a waiting list of men who wanted to be her date for dinner that night (yes, you read it right—she insisted that all men who wanted to date her should send her an official request through the internal mail service and then she would send a response back by mail to the chosen gentleman), getting dressed with care, waiting in her room for the chosen gentleman to escort her to dinner, waltzing for a few minutes after dinner and going back to her room to sleep. When I wanted to visit her for her routine checkup, I had to send her a request letter and wait for her to fit me into her busy schedule. If I showed up late she would refuse to see me, and if I showed up early she made me wait until our appointment time. And often I had to wait a long time for her.

During one of my visits to her she turned to me and said, "Dr. Ayati, why don't you just write a book about all the medical tips and advice you keep giving me and send it to me. I will read it when I can, and in this way I don't have to fit you into my busy schedule. I am not getting any younger and really don't have time for these visits from you any longer."

I have finally taken her advice. My visits with her brought a lot of pleasure and enthusiasm for me and were the highlights of my days. God bless her soul, she knew how to live, play and enjoy life to the fullest. She did not let anything get in her way. That is how we should all live.

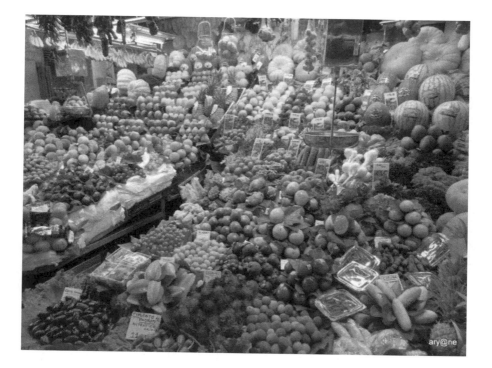

Chapter 1

Nutrition

Questions To Ask Yourself

At the beginning of each chapter, including this one, you will find a set of questions relating the chapter theme to your current health situation and practices. Take time to think about each one and answer it as thoroughly and honestly as you can.

1. Are you losing any weight (voluntarily or involuntarily)? How much weight have you lost in the past year? List the reason(s) why you have lost weight (low appetite, depression, illness, etc.).

2. Do you take any vitamins, supplements, herbal remedies or prescription drugs?

3. Do you follow any specific diet (vegan, vegetarian, protein, carbohydrate, fat, Mediterranean diet, etc.)? Why do you follow this diet (health concerns, religious beliefs, media pressure, etc.)? Are you obsessed with your weight?

4. What do you eat? List everything you eat regularly in a week (vegetables, fruits, meats, sweets, grains, etc.)?

5. What do you drink (water, juices, coffee, tea, alcohol, etc.) in a day? List everything you drink and the amount of each.

6. Do you see a dentist regularly? How often (every six months)?

7. How many social activities are you engaged in?

A few years back a healthy middle aged man walked into my clinic and asked for a prescription to lose weight. He mentioned that he had gone through a recent divorce and was once again in the dating market. He thought that the weight loss would make him feel more confident and competitive and also make him healthier. When I told him that he did not need to lose weight and could achieve the same results by engaging in a moderate level of exercise he accused me of siding with his ex-wife and started throwing profanity at me. He was kindly asked to leave the clinic! He then called my clinic's manager and asked for a refund. He complained that I refused to prescribe him a weight loss medication even though his insurance was fully charged for the visit. And of course the refund was not granted.

Nutrition and diet are two major areas of concern for the elderly as well as the general population. In my practice I am continuously faced with the following questions:

- I have lost my appetite and am losing weight. Could you give me an appetite stimulant?
- I eat well, but I can't gain any weight. What should I do?
- Why am I losing weight?
- Why am I gaining weight?
- What should I do to lose weight? Should I take an appetite suppressant?
- What's the best diet?
- Should I take any supplements? Vitamins? Herbal remedies?

3

Many of my patients have put themselves through various types of diets in order to lose or gain weight. It's no surprise— they are constantly bombarded by the media, magazine articles, books, and even the scientific community to follow specific diets, such as the carbohydrate diet, fat diet, protein diet, vegetarian diet, vegan, the Mediterranean, etc., for better health and longer life. In most cases, these diets have proven unbeneficial for them, and all too often they have ended up in even worse health.

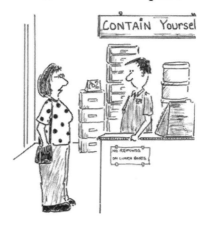

"I need something that will hold two dozen diet books, kindling, and a starter log."

And it's not just diets—many of my patients are looking for the best supplement that could act as a magic solution for better health. Sadly, this unfounded belief in the power of supplements has become a practice model in our society. Most of the patients admitted into skilled nursing facilities and hospitals today come with an order of multivitamins. And all too often when a patient is at a hospital or skilled nursing facility, and losing weight, the first action is adding protein and calorie supplements like Ensure. Although sometimes it is necessary to give sick and critically ill patients supplemental calories, this has unfortunately become a general practice. In some countries it is even normal practice for the physicians to infuse their patients with vitamin B12 and

B-Complex on a monthly basis! I have actually had patients walk out of my clinic when I refused to prescribe unnecessary supplements to them or told them to stop taking the ones they were taking.

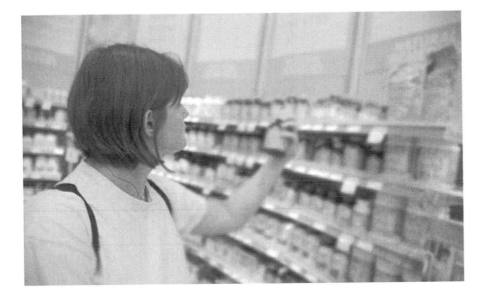

Proper diet and nutrition are essential factors for health, and unfortunately, drastic diets, supplements, and appetite stimulants or suppressants do not address and resolve weight loss or gain issues. In order to understand this concept we need to talk about the physiological processes that take place in our body as we age. But first let me explain why as a geriatrician I am very sensitive to detecting weight loss and in immediately addressing the underlying cause.

It is more alarming to me when my patients or their family members report weight loss--more alarming than if they are overweight, have high blood pressure or uncontrolled blood sugar levels! Scientific studies tell us that weight loss in older adults is associated with an increased rate of disease and death. Data indicate that even the loss of a small percent of weight over a three-year period is associated with multiple negative health outcomes such as frailty, fatigue, a higher risk of infection, delirium (confusion) and an increased death rate in the elderly.[1,2]

The Causes of Weight Loss in The Elderly

When your body ages, your physical activities tend to decrease and you lose bone mass, muscles and water content while increasing fat content. Along with these changes, your metabolism decreases. This results in a reduction in your total energy expenditure and a decrease in appetite. What can you do to counter that? You need to increase your energy expenditure by exercising moderately and increasing your normal physical activity. This will result in building new muscles and decreasing your percentage of body fat. As a result you will see an increase in your appetite and normal weight gain if you eat a healthy diet. This process will also help to decrease your blood pressure and control diabetes and arthritis if you have them. We will read more about the right kind of physical activity and exercise in future chapters.

In addition to the physiological role of weight loss there are other factors that can contribute to it.

1. **As we age we lose our taste buds.** If you have ever taken cold lozenges packed with zinc, you have surely noticed that you can't taste food properly for a few hours to a day afterward. Everything tastes like cardboard! You lose your appetite and don't want to eat. A similar process occurs as you age. To compensate for the loss of taste buds you might find yourself adding more salt to your food—that can increase your blood pressure. Besides your taste, your sense of smell also declines with age.

   One way to counter this loss is to work on the food presentation. Food becomes more palatable when you add bright colored vegetables and fruits to your plate or serve the food in colorful dishes or your best china. After all, as the French say, we eat with our eyes first. Unfortunately, most senior care facilities, hospitals, assisted-living communities, and charitable home-delivered meal services offer truly boring food. Needless to say the presentation is also lacking.

   The quality of the food you serve is of utmost importance. Foods (preferably organic if available) free of preservatives, herbicides, pesticides, hormones, and antibiotics can taste better. Try to limit your intake of foods that come out of a can or the freezer compartment of your grocery store, especially those containing high levels of salt. Weather permitting,

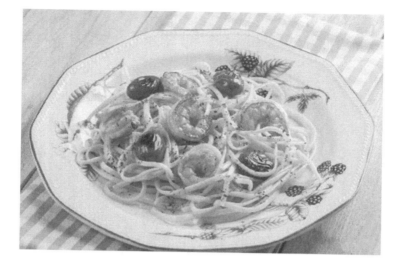

try to eat local seasonal produce bought from your farmer's market. Shopping this way helps you with your physical activity and also allows you to build meaningful relationships. My parents know their produce merchant, butcher, baker, and fishermen on a first name basis. They have made buying their food into a pleasant ritual. They enjoy socializing and interacting with their community while shopping for their everyday meal.

I was in Cinque Terre on the Italian Riviera with my wife a few years back. Twice a day the elders there do a ritual walk up and down the narrow, steep streets. They talk to their neighbors, gossip, learn about the latest news and do their daily shopping. They socialize, get fresh air, feel a valuable part of their community and get all the exercise their bodies need. Therefore, when people say the Mediterranean diet is

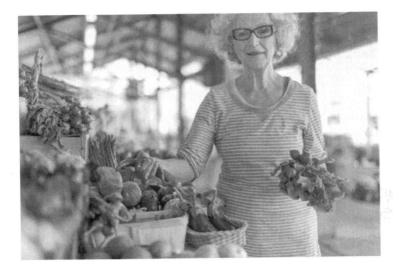

good for you, I say the whole experience just described is even better. You can sit in an apartment by yourself and eat fish and olives and drink the best wine, but you will not benefit as much.

2. **As we age we are prone to losing our teeth.** During a recent visit back home, I noticed that my father had lost a lot of weight. Naturally, I became alarmed and started investigating the root cause. It turned out that his teeth were the problem-- he had lost so many of them that he was unable to chew his food. As a result he ate less (especially fresh fruits, vegetables and meats), started having gastrointestinal issues (such as bloating, belching, gas, indigestion, abdominal pain, nausea, etc.), and was not the normal social butterfly I knew. He felt embarrassed to eat in front of others. And he felt helpless since his friends who had dentures told him

they could not enjoy most foods, and therefore, he thought they were not a viable solution. A visit to the dentist did wonders—following a consultation, he decided to get dental implants. Along with other modern options, dental implants are a relatively painless solution and mostly affordable in many countries. An exception is the US, where, depending on the practice you choose, implants can be an expensive procedure and not affordable by most seniors since they are often not covered by insurance. In such case talk to your dentist about the new generation dentures. I have many patients who use them and are fairly satisfied with them. Also, visit your dentist every six months and make sure you have no gum inflammation or tooth infections. Dental and gum issues can lead to heart and kidney disease.

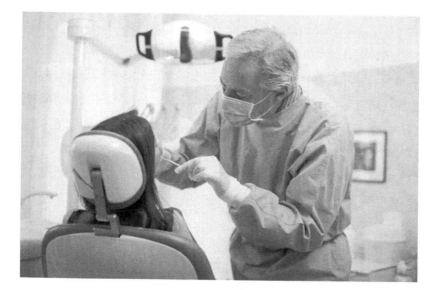

Another issue to keep in mind is that patients suffering from chronic arthritis can develop pain in the jaw, specifically in the temporomandibular (TM) joint that attaches the jaw to the skull. This sometimes manifests itself as a headache, and it can also interfere with chewing food. A painless injection of cortisone into the TM joint, prescribed by a doctor, can often relieve the pain and treat the problem.

3. **Lack of access to transportation**. In countries such as the US, where people may live miles away from shopping centers and have very poor public transportation infrastructure, getting around is a major issue for many elderly. Many don't drive and are dependent on others for their everyday shopping excursions. Because of this, the majority get their nutrition from canned or frozen pre-cooked meals bought in large quantities. As mentioned, these foods can be very low in quality and are often packed with preservatives and salt. They should be avoided as much as possible. However, if they are the only available option make sure to read the labels on the packaging and choose the ones lowest in salt and sugar, and ideally free of preservatives. If the labels are too long and full of ingredients you do not recognize, it is best to avoid them.

Instead of buying canned or frozen food, try buying enough fresh vegetables, eggs, and yogurt to last in your refrigerator for a couple of weeks. Buy good quality (preferably organic, grass fed) chicken, lamb, pork, beef, or wild fish (those low in mercury), or farm fish free of antibiotics and hormones and store them in your freezer for up to six months. Instead of salt, try adding herbs such as dried/fresh dill, oregano, tarragon, basil, cilantro, rosemary, etc. to your food. Herbs have strong aromatic oils, which add a lot of flavor and zest to your food. To avoid cooking every day make a large pot of food with your fresh ingredients and it can last in your refrigerator for up to a week (with the exception of fish, which should be consumed as soon as possible to avoid bacterial infections). Slow cookers and Dutch ovens are all very helpful too. You can put your vegetables, some herbs and a piece of meat in one and let it slowly cook your food to perfection. What is great is that you do not need to check it every few minutes. And the food tastes delicious in slow cookers. Together with my wife, we try this often as we both have hectic schedules.

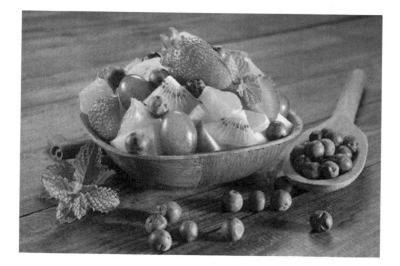

Buy lots of seasonal fruits. Avoid refrigerating them when you can since fruits stored in the refrigerator can taste awful. Refrigeration slows fruit ripening. Therefore, if fruits are harvested prior to being ripened it is important to store them at room temperature without moving them to your refrigerator until they are fully ripe. Unripened fruits exposed to cold temperatures can suffer internal breakdown, which may result in flavorless taste. Leave them in a colorful basket on your kitchen table and help yourself to them. If too many of them ripen at the same time put them in a fruit salad or a regular salad and enjoy them. If you do not have nut allergies, enjoy a handful of them as snacks. Always have a nice bottle of extra virgin olive oil on hand. It tastes fruity, nutty and stimulates your tastes buds. You can add it to your salads and vegetables, brush it on your toast instead of butter

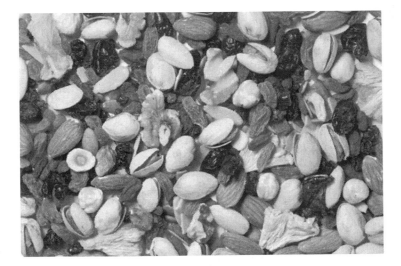

(which contains cholesterol and high levels of saturated fat), and cook with it. Olive oil contains monounsaturated fatty acids that can lower your risk of heart disease. And remember to consume all foods, even the healthiest ones, in moderation.

4. **Lack of companionship**. Imagine after all the years of preparing and eating your meals with family, friends and colleagues you now have to eat alone—meal after meal. Many elderly who are retired, have lost a spouse, or are far away from their busy children and other family members have to face this every day.

It is imperative to create meaningful relationships at any age, but even more so as we get older. Volunteering for the many different social institutions and programs (kindergartens, schools, hospitals, libraries, public radio, food drives,

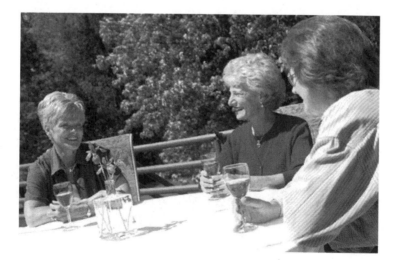

etc.), becoming a mentor to a young child, and participating in or organizing cultural, religious or scholarly events are a few of the many ways to find companions and form meaningful connections. I have noticed that in many assisted living communities people eat in front of their TV alone in their room. Force yourself to move out of your room and into the society. It is just like networking. The first few encounters might be hard but then you get the hang of it.

My father-in-law lives a few months a year in Iran and the rest of the year in Canada and the US. In Iran he lives alone. For a few consecutive years, every time he visited us in the US we noticed that he had lost weight and looked pale and frail. We asked him why, and he said he hated eating lunches alone and often ended up skipping lunch altogether. He did not feel like cooking lunches for only himself either. However, when he was with us in the US he ate well and gained weight. He was healthy and in very good spirits at the end of his visits. We kept encouraging him to socialize with people and eat in good company while he was in Iran.

Lunch time in Iran is a very sacred, peaceful and personal event as opposed to supper, which is a time shared with friends and family. You eat your lunch with your immediate family (mostly at home) and then take a nap. With no family at home and no other close companion, he adjusted by simply avoiding lunch, with unhealthy consequences. Finally, he seems to have heeded our advice—this year he told us that he found a great companion. He is now eating his lunches with the owner of a local grocery store in his neighborhood. In Iran people buy their daily groceries from their local stores. My dad has been buying his daily groceries from this gentleman for years. The store owner had recently lost his spouse and was similarly having a very difficult time. My father-in-law offered to cook for the two of them every day while this gentleman provided the fresh ingredients. They developed the habit of eating their lunches together, discussing the price of grains, the economy, the old neighborhood, their children and politics. Now, both are thriving again. If you or one of your loved ones is elderly and regularly eating alone, it would be wise to follow their lead and look for some mealtime companionship.

A related issue I have often encountered is that once an elderly patient loses a spouse or partner, the survivor faces devastation, despair, isolation, anxiety and depression. Losing a source of companionship, support and stability is indeed a tragedy. Studies have indicated that the death or illness of a spouse increases the mortality rate for the survivor by 21 percent for a husband and by 17 percent for a wife.[3] While you might find yourself alone in such tragic situations, you should dedicate yourself to adapting over time in order to arrive at a level of physical, emotional and psychological stability. You can recover much faster by keeping busy. Encircle yourself with new or old friends and family members, and draw support from your community. Exercise, meditate, travel, volunteer, resume work or find a part-time job, and date. Yes, date. Although many of my patients and their children find the notion of dating shocking, inappropriate and distressing, I encourage my single patients to actively look for a partner. There is no shame or guilt in wanting to find love and a companion to share life with. While it is delightful to have the companionship of friends and family members it still gets lonely at the end of the day.

5. **Financial hardship.** The sad reality is that a large number of seniors are living in poverty in the US as well as abroad. The recent global economic crisis of 2008, the collapse of the housing market and the astronomically high cost of healthcare in the US are among the many factors contributing to the growth of debt among the elderly. Some of them are forced to forgo retirement and seek very low paying jobs, which they may still have a very hard time finding due to age discrimination. They may be faced with a hard choice between paying their mortgage for a roof over their head, buying the many medications they can't survive without, or purchasing food. Often food is the last thing on their mind. While this problem is somewhat contained in Canada and many European countries with socialized healthcare, the elderly still have their socioeconomic challenges. And indeed this is a very hard problem to tackle.

A few years back I had a very kind, proud and respectable patient on Medicare. She lived in an old house with her grandson. She had many medical issues and had been in an out of hospitals and nursing homes for years. The plumbing and heating systems in her house were ancient and didn't work well. They could not warm themselves in the winter and were unable to take showers. And she was malnourished. She felt ashamed and desolate. Her grandson was attending school, already working part time, and doing his best to take care of her, but they still could not make ends meet. Repeatedly, she would ask me if she could skip her medications as she could not afford them. Food was the last thing on her mind. I referred her to social services, but unfortunately, she passed away before they were able to help her. It was heartbreaking and a very common situation among the elderly.

If you are wealthy, thank your lucky stars and share with those unfortunate seniors in need of financial help. It will be very rewarding for you and you will form meaningful and spiritual relationships in the process. If you have difficulty buying food, ask your physicians or social workers for help. They can refer you to food banks or help you get food stamps. There are many organizations out there ready to offer help, and there is no shame in seeking it.

6. **Medical issues and stress.** Medical conditions and stress can result in a loss of appetite and hence weight loss. As we age there is an accumulation of molecular, cellular, and or-

gan damage within our body. Physiological and environmental factors (pollution, herbicides, pesticides, etc.) put us
at a higher risk of developing chronic diseases and cancer.
Diabetes, arthritis, cardiovascular disease, hypertension,
dementia (including Alzheimer's), depression, kidney and
bladder problems, Parkinson's, lung disease (especially if
you have been or are a smoker), cataracts, glaucoma, mac-
ular degeneration, osteoporosis, and enlarged prostate are
a few of these chronic diseases. Seniors dealing with any of
these diseases are taking multiple medications and are suffering from varying degree of pain. Most medications such
as antidepressants, pain relievers and those prescribed for
cardiac problems cause loss of appetite.

Psychological factors also play a role in weight loss. When
seniors suffer from increased stress and anxiety, they can experience fatigue, depression and loss of appetite. Often, they
feel helpless as they believe they are losing control as well as
their freedom and autonomy. Keep in mind that sometimes
what could seem to be a psychological factor contributing
to weight loss can in fact be due to an underlying medical
reason. A clinician I once worked with told me a story about
a friend of hers, Maggie, who lost twenty pounds in a very
short period of time. Maggie normally weighed around a
hundred pounds and was very concerned when she lost a
large amount of weight in just a few months. She saw her
primary care physician who insisted the weight loss was due

to stress and referred her to a nutritionist without follow up. Luckily, Maggie was not convinced by the diagnosis and got a second opinion from another physician. The second physician ran some tests and unfortunately Maggie was diagnosed with breast cancer, which had metastasized to other organs in her body. Fortunately, Maggie was referred to an oncologist, and after an intense course of treatment is now cancer free.

Gastrointestinal issues are also very common as we age. Slow bowel movements, constipation, irritable bowel syndrome, maldigestion (the inability to absorb nutrients) and slow gastric emptying give us a sensation of fullness and bloating. You might wonder about gastric emptying. When you eat, the food stays in your stomach for an average of half an hour before it is released into the small intestine. However, this interval increases with age, and because the food stays in your stomach for a longer period of time, you experience early satiety after eating a small portion of food. Therefore, you might have a great appetite but after taking a few bites you feel full and unable to eat more.[4] The key in this case is to have more frequent meals but eat less at each.

Many of these conditions can be avoided through preventative measures. Therefore, make sure to visit your primary care doctor routinely and your geriatrician at least once a year. A lot of patients have confided in me about being afraid of doctors and avoiding checkups until it is too late. They say they are terrified of what they might find wrong with their bodies. Although this may be understandable at an emotional level, it really doesn't make sense. Would you drive your car indefinitely without any oil change or checkups? Then your body, which is the most precious element of your life, should be treated with the utmost care and diligence. Early detection is crucial. We are lucky to live in an era when advanced diagnostic tools allow the very early detection of a number of diseases. And if diseases are diagnosed early, advancements in the fields of medicine and biotechnology enable a good prognosis in many cases. Finding out that you have a serious disease is depressing, but finding out you have a serious disease that has become less treatable or even untreatable because you waited is devastating. It is much better to be tested and diagnosed early so that you can start the necessary treatment as soon as possible.

If you suffer from any of these conditions, do not despair. You can still have a comfortable life ahead. Erroneously, we have been programed to be terrified of the words *chronic disease* and *cancer*. Even people suffering from cancer can now live for many years. The best thing is to correctly inform yourself (via your doctor, the Internet, books & literature, associated foundations, support groups, etc.) about your condition. The more you know, the better you can prepare yourself to live a high quality and independent life. Nowadays technology advancements (such as reminder and safety devices or services, automatic lifts, kitchen, bathroom, and walking gadgets, etc.) allow people to age and take care of themselves in the comfort of their home, inexpensively. Most of our fear and anxiety come from the unknown. The sooner you close that chapter the better off you will be. When faced with a serious illness or condition, understand it and manage it—don't let it manage you.

What Should I Eat?

Having talked about the many reasons underlying weight and appetite loss in the elderly I will now discuss a few healthy habits and key nutrients for optimal health. You might remember that in the late eighties the media was telling us to eat a diet full of carbohydrates and stay away from fat by all means. Fat became the enemy and people stuffed themselves with pastas and breads. Diet drinks and foods loaded with chemicals became very popular. You may also remember that following this diet, the overall population put on a lot of weight and became more diabetic and sicker than ever. Our body uses carbohydrates as fuel. However, if we eat too much (in excess of what is needed as fuel) our body converts them into fat.

In the nineties the fat and protein diet became very popular. The media stated that now the carbohydrates were the enemies, while fat and proteins were good for us. We were encouraged to eat butter, cheese, fatty meats and stay away from carbohydrates. That did not work either. Although some individuals had success, overall we did not lose weight and our health continued to go downward. Too much fat and protein put our cardiovascular and renal systems in shock, respectively.

In the early 2000s vegetarian and vegan diets became very fashionable. Now fat, meats, and carbohydrates were the enemies and fiber was in. While fiber is necessary for gastrointestinal health, too much of it is unhealthy. I see many patients in my clinic with severe gastrointestinal problems (constipation, bloating, belching, pain, etc.) who are taking massive amounts of fiber. Since 2010 the Mediterranean diet has become popular. Drink red wine every night and load yourself with olive oil, nuts and fish (which could be full of mercury if it is wild and hormones and antibiotics if it is farm-raised).

Let me stop here. Exaggeration does not work. Each of these key nutrients plays a vital role in our physiology. For example, our body needs carbohydrates for fuel, fat for memory and the nervous system, protein to build muscles, and a moderate amount of fiber for our gastrointestinal system to function smoothly. The best practice is to eat a range of foods that are healthy and that you enjoy. And remember that even the healthiest balanced diet can lead to weight gain if too much is consumed. Therefore, moderation is the key. Don't follow fad diets. History has shown us over and over that they can be harmful for your body and your mental health.

Unless you suffer from a specific medical illness that indicates otherwise, your diet should be composed of 20-35 % fat, 45-65 % carbohydrates and 10-35 % protein. This ratio may need to be changed based on your health condition. For example, if you suffer from heart disease or high cholesterol you may need to decrease the amount of saturated, trans-fatty acid and total cholesterol. Instead you may need to take more unsaturated fats or foods enriched with high density lipoprotein (HDL) like olive oil, canola or fish oil. Keep in mind that certain types of wild fish (such as tuna) could have high levels of mercury (for more information check this website: http://www.nrdc.org/health/effects/mercury/guide.asp). Mercury is poisonous and affects the gastrointestinal, renal and neurological systems. Therefore, do not load yourself with fish oil supplements! Another very important word of advice is not to cut fat from your diet entirely. Our body needs fat to function properly. As mentioned above, our brain and nervous system are also dependent on fat to function and repair themselves properly.

Here are a few other things to keep in mind:

- **Hydration.** If you do not suffer from congestive heart failure, liver disease (especially cirrhosis) and other medical conditions resulting in fluid overload, hydration is of utmost importance. On average, your fluid intake should be 30 ml (approximately 1 oz.) per kg (each kg is 2.2 pounds) of body weight. For example, if you are 70 kg, you need 70 x

30= 2,100 ml (about 2 liters) of fluid per day. While all fluids count toward the daily total, it is best to drink water and limit sugary or sugar free sodas, juices, or tea and coffee beverages. Keep in mind that as we age we lose our thirst sensation and as such we do not feel thirsty as often. Therefore, make sure to hydrate yourself even if you do not feel thirsty. Furthermore, the amount of a hormone called ADH (Anti-Diuretic Hormone) released from our brain subsides with age. This hormone travels from the brain via blood to the kidneys and increases water absorption. As such, our body produces less urine when the outside temperature increases or when we exercise and do not hydrate ourselves adequately. However, if our body does not produce enough ADH (which is the case as our body ages) we will get dehydrated fast. This is the most common cause of ER visits for the elderly and if not addressed properly can lead to death. Remind yourself (either by the help of technology gadgets such as phone, alarms, reminder services, etc.) or ask your family members to remind you to drink enough fluid on a daily basis. But keep in mind not to exaggerate either. Don't drink yourself to death!

- **Vitamin D and other vitamins.** I am sure you have heard a lot on the topic of vitamin D from the media and possibly from your doctors. Recent studies are very controversial about the benefits, proper dosage and side effects of vitamin D. Let me give you a brief and simple biochemistry lesson on vitamins here to help you understand them better.

Our body utilizes two categories of vitamins: water soluble and fat soluble. The water soluble group includes vitamins such as B and C. Our body requires a certain amount of these vitamins to function properly. If you take in more than what the normal physiological level should be, the extra amount is simply excreted from your body (via urine). Therefore, while water soluble vitamins do not harm you if taken in excess, they do not provide any extra benefit. As such, you do not need a shot of vitamin B12 every month unless if a physician has determined from your routine blood test results that you are deficient. The same thing is true with vitamin C. There is no demonstrated benefit in taking extra amounts of vitamin C on a daily basis.

The second group of vitamins includes the fat soluble ones such as vitamins A, K, E, and D. If these are taken in extra amounts, the body cannot excrete the excess. Consequently, they can actually reach toxic levels in the body and be very harmful. For example, vitamin D is necessary for the absorption of calcium in our body. If taken in excess, your blood calcium increases and you will be at a higher risk of experiencing constipation, abdominal pain, anxiety, kidney stones, bone pain, and other adverse health conditions.

As mentioned above, the role of Vitamin D is to increase absorption of calcium from our gastrointestinal system. Calcium is the building block of bones, in addition to being necessary for many other physiological functions in our body. It is crucial for us to get enough calcium and vitamin D to prevent weakening of the bones—a condition called osteoporosis, which can result in bone fractures and curvature. A small number of studies have shown the effect of Vitamin D in improving leg strength, reducing the risk of falls[5,6] and reducing colon cancer.[7,8] There have also been data indicating that vitamin D deficiency can result in diabetes, cardiovascular disease, hypertension and obesity.[9] However, these results are very limited and inconclusive.

On the other hand, a recent study by the National Cancer Institute has indicated the possibility of an increased risk of pancreatic cancer in people taking high levels of vitamin D.[10] Therefore, we go back to the common theme in this chapter. Moderation is the key. Just because one study indicates some benefits from taking vitamin D, that is not enough to justify taking massive doses of it.

To find out whether your vitamin D level is normal, your doctor needs to order a simple blood test. The normal range of vitamin D (25-hydroxy vitamin D) is between 30.0 to 74.0 nanograms per milliliter (ng/ml). If your blood vitamin D level is low, your doctor can prescribe dietary supplements for you. However, make sure to follow up with your doctor periodically (at least every three months) to see if your vitamin D level has normalized and do not continue to take vitamin D supplements indefinitely. The amount of vitamin D intake per day (from food or supplements) should be 800 international units (IUs) for seniors (ages 71 and older) and 600 IUs for anyone younger. Vitamin D must be taken together with calcium to maintain strong bones. The recommended daily level of calcium for seniors is 1,200 mg.

If you do not have any liver, kidney, or gastrointestinal diseases and are not taking certain medications (such as phenytoin, phenobarbital, and rifampin), you should be able to get enough calcium and vitamin D from your diet. In the US, most dairy products, breads, and non-dairy beverages such as rice milk and almond milk are fortified with vitamin D and calcium. Our body can also synthesize vitamin D from cholesterol when our skin gets adequate sun exposure. Therefore, make sure to have a limited amount of sun exposure every day. Moderation is key again. Don't burn yourself and increase your risk of getting skin cancer. Your skin color, the season, the length and time of day, the level of air pollution and cloud levels are among the factors that can affect the amount of sun exposure you might need: for more information refer to: http://ods.od.nih.gov/factsheets/VitaminD-HealthProfessional/. For most people, just a short walk of about 30 minutes a day in the sun between 10 AM and 3 PM should do it. And you will need to have an adequate level of cholesterol for this process. Hence, unlike what you may have seen or heard in the media, cholesterol, once more in moderation, is not the enemy.

Let us briefly discuss other vitamins. Most of our processed food in the U.S is fortified with vitamins. In addition, the majority of the population is currently taking multivitamin and mineral supplements on a daily basis. They are under the assumption that these vitamins keep them healthy and energetic. However most of studies done so far do not support this. The role of multivitamin and mineral supplements in preventing chronic diseases and infections was discussed in detail at the National Institute of Health (NIH) conference in 2006 and addressed by recent publications.[11-13] Studies showed that supplements do not boost immunity against infections such as pneumonia or urine infection and do not prevent cancer or cardiovascular disease. And some vitamins and supplements can even result in adverse health effects. For example, smokers taking Beta Carotene (vitamin A) are at a higher risk of cancer. Furthermore, as you will see from the Overmedication chapter in this book, vitamins can interfere with prescription drugs and cause neuropathy, organ damage and even death. They can also counter the effect of your medications. For instance, vitamin K can reverse the effect of Warfarin (a blood thinner, also called Coumadin). Hence, if you are not deficient in vitamins and minerals, it is not beneficial to take dietary supplements. The bottom line: *Get your vitamins from food rather than supplements.*

Note that if you are taking medications, always check with your doctor about the kinds of food you should avoid. As mentioned, you can get your vitamins from food. However, sometimes the vitamins you absorb from your food can also reverse the effect of the medications you take. For example, if you are taking blood thinners you should avoid eating leafy greens as they contain vitamin K, which as we saw counters the effect of that class of drugs.

What About Being Overweight?

For adults a body mass index (BMI) less than 18.5 is considered underweight, while a BMI between 25 and 29.9 is considered overweight and a BMI of 30 or higher is considered obese (for more information refer to http://www.cdc.gov/obesity/adult/defining.html). BMI is calculated by using weight and height of individuals and, *for most people*, it correlates with their amount of body fat. Most people, however, erroneously correlate being overweight or obese with a higher risk of developing diseases. It is crucial to keep in mind that for assessing someone's likelihood of developing overweight- or obesity-related diseases (such as cardiovascular disease, high blood pressure, type 2 diabetes, and certain cancers) three key factors are considered:

1. BMI
2. Waist circumference: The higher an individual's waist circumference (which means a higher abdominal fat content)

the higher is her or his risk of developing heart disease and type 2 diabetes. Normal waist size for women is less than 35 inches and for men less than 40 inches.

3. Risk factors for developing cardiovascular disease: These are factors such as high blood pressure, high level of bad cholesterol (called LDL), low level of good cholesterol (called HDL), high triglycerides, high blood sugar, family history of heart disease, physical inactivity and smoking.

Therefore, people who are overweight but do not have a high waist measurement and have fewer than two risk factors are not at a higher risk of developing diseases. During your routine annual checkups your physician can determine if you are at an increased risk by evaluating your BMI, waist measurement, and other risk factors for heart disease. If your physician determines that you are at risk you should increase your physical activity and seek a nutritionist's advice on how to *slowly* (and let me emphasize the word *slowly*) lose weight.

At the beginning of this chapter I mentioned that as a geriatrician, I am more concerned if a patient is losing weight rather than being overweight due to the risks mentioned. However, I know a lot of patients are worried about being overweight, as are their families. Let me briefly discuss a few points about patients who are overweight. Recent studies have indicated that people who are overweight have a longer life expectancy compared to people who are obese, are underweight or have a normal weight.

[14-16] These studies were somewhat surprising but at some level logical. One of the theories behind this is that as we age we are more prone to developing chronic diseases, infectious diseases (such as pneumonia), and cancer as well as undergoing more surgeries. The elderly who suffer from these conditions are at a higher risk of losing weight and experiencing frailty (more on this in the chapter on Frailty) and as a result having an increased death rate. Therefore, being overweight gives them a sort of a "cushion". For instance, fat tissues provide the higher energy required for the healing process. Furthermore, it turns out that hormones produced from fat have anti-inflammatory properties, which aid with the recovery. Another theory is that overweight people might seek better medical care and get screened more regularly for chronic diseases compared to those with normal weight. Also, doctors tend to treat their overweight patients more aggressively.

We have learned in this chapter that as we age we become less physically active. Our metabolism decreases, and we lose our muscles and increase our fat content. Increasing our physical activity and eating a balanced diet should help us maintain a healthy weight. My advice is therefore not to be obsessed with your weight but rather concentrate on enjoying life, decreasing your stress level, and pursuing your interests. Make sure to visit your physician for routine checkups.

Take Home Message

The common theme in this chapter is moderation. Avoid drastic diets, especially jumping into the current fads. Eat nutritious foods in small portions but more frequently and in good company. Practice "mindful eating". This means slowing down and appreciating things like the sights, smells, textures, and tastes of your food as you eat. Chew your food slowly and thoroughly. And get rid of distractions such as your cell phone, computer, TV, work assignments, emails, etc. It has been proposed that mindful eating could alleviate stress as well as chronic gastrointestinal problems and high blood pressure (for more information refer to: http://tinyurl.com/6fjjx3j). Supplements and vitamins should be avoided unless if your doctor has detected low levels of them in your routine blood test. Moderate activity will help you maintain a healthy weight.

ACTION PLAN

Now that you have read this chapter go back to the questionnaire at the beginning of this chapter and review your answers. Discuss them with your physician during your next appointment. Can you change any of your habits? Do this for the future chapters as well.

1. Make a list of social activities of interest and sign up for them

2. Make an appointment with your dentist

3. If you have unintentionally lost more than 5% of your body weight in one year list the reason(s) why you have lost weight (low appetite, depression, illness, etc.) and discuss this with your physician as soon as possible

4. Make sure to eat healthy food in good company at least once a week

5. Make a list of all you eat and drink in one week and see if you can improve your diet

6. If you take any vitamins, supplements, herbal remedies or any prescription drugs list all of them (with the dosage per day) and the reason why you are taking each and show the list to your physician

REFERENCES

1. Reasons for intentional weight loss, unintentional weight loss, and mortality in older men. Wannamethee SG, Shaper AG, Lennon L, Arch Intern Med. 2005;165(9):1035.

2. Weight change in old age and its association with mortality. Newman AB, Yanez D, Harris T, Duxbury A, Enright PL, Fried LP, Cardiovascular Study Research Group, J Am Geriatric Soc. 2001;49(10):1309.

3. Mortality after the Hospitalization of a Spouse. Christakis NA, and Allison PD, N Engl J Med 2006; 354:719-730.

4. Changes in gastric emptying rates with age. Horowitz M, Maddern GJ, Chatterton BE, Collins PJ, Harding PE, Shearman D, JClin Sci (Lond). 1984;67(2):213.

5. Fall risk and fracture. Vitamin D and falls/fractures. Miyakoshi N, Clin Calcium. 2013;23(5):695-700.

6. Fall prevention in community-dwelling older adults. Robertson MC, Gillespie LD, JAMA. 2013;309(13):1406-7.

7. Vitamin D3 insufficiency and colorectal cancer. Di Rosa M, Malaguarnera M, Zanchì A, Passaniti A, Malaguarnera L, Crit Rev Oncol Hematol. 2013;pii: S1040-8428(13)00167-4.

8. Association between vitamin D and risk of colorectal cancer: a systematic review of prospective studies. Ma Y, Zhang P, Wang F, Yang J, Liu Z, Qin H, J Clin Oncol. 2011;29(28):3775-82.

9. The impact of vitamin D deficiency on diabetes and cardiovascular risk. Baz-Hecht M, Goldfine AB, Curr Opin Endocrinol Diabetes Obes. 2010;17(2):113-9.

10. Circulating 25-hydroxyvitamin D and risk of pancreatic cancer: Cohort Consortium Vitamin D Pooling Project of Rarer Cancers. Stolzenberg-Solomon RZ, Jacobs EJ, Arslan AA, Qi D, Patel AV, Helzlsouer KJ, Weinstein SJ, McCullough ML, Purdue MP, Shu XO, Snyder K, Virtamo J,Wilkins LR, Yu K, Zeleniuch-Jacquotte A, Zheng W, Albanes D, Cai Q, Harvey C, Hayes R, Clipp S, Horst RL, Irish L, Koenig K, Le Marchand L, Kolonel LN, Am J Epidemiol. 2010;172(1):81-93.

11. National Institutes of Health State-of-the-science conference statement: multivitamin/mineral supplements and chronic disease prevention. NIH State-of-the-Science Panel, Ann Intern Med. 2006;145(5):364.

12. Enough is enough: Stop wasting money on vitamin and mineral supplements. Guallar E, Stranges S, Mulrow C, Appel LJ, Miller ER 3rd, Ann Intern Med. 2013;159(12):850-1.

13. Vitamin, Mineral, and Multivitamin Supplements for the Primary Prevention of Cardiovascular Disease and Cancer: U.S. Preventive Services Task Force Recommendation Statement. Moyer VA, Ann Intern Med. 2014 Feb 25.

14. Association of all-cause mortality with overweight and obesity using standard body mass index categories: a systematic review and meta-analysis. Flegal KM, Kit BK, Orpana H, Graubard BI, JAMA. 2013;309(1):71-82.

15. Body composition and mortality risk in later life. Toss F, Wiklund P, Nordström P, Nordström A, Age Ageing. 2012;41(5):677-81.

16. Population heterogeneity in the impact of body weight on mortality. Zheng H, Yang Y, Soc Sci Med. 2012;75(6):990-6.

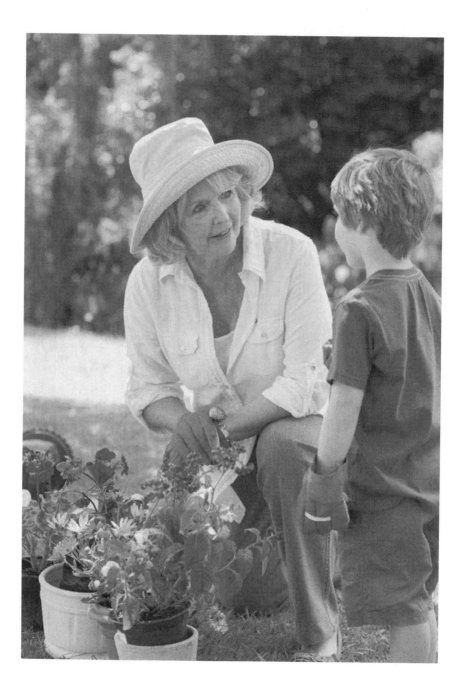

Chapter 2

Mental Health

Questions to Ask Yourself

1. Do you enjoy your life? Is there anything you would like to change?

2. Are you a happy person? Do you surround yourself with happy, positive people and cheerful ambiances?

3. Do you have any hobbies?

4. Are there any new activities you would like to try?

5. Do you suffer from depression, anxiety, memory loss, etc.? If so, do you see your physician regularly?

6. Write down the list of all the medications you are taking including any anti-depressants, anti-anxiety medications, vitamins, supplements, or herbal remedies. Show the list to your physician and make sure it is OK to take them.

7. Do you exercise regularly? If not, write down the reason(s) why you do not wish to exercise or why you are unable to exercise. Share this with your physician.

8. Do you exercise obsessively? If so, have you discussed this with your physician?

9. Do you have a good appetite and eat a healthy balanced diet? If not, explain why you think you have low appetite and make sure to discuss this with your physician.

10. Do you have a good support system (from family members, friends, your community, etc.)? If not, what might you do to improve it?

11. What is the level of your social engagement? Do you interact with your community? Do you do any volunteer work? Do you belong to any club(s)?

12. Do you meditate (religiously or spiritually)?

13. What are your cholesterol and blood pressure levels? Do you take any medications for high cholesterol and high blood pressure levels? Discuss these with your physician.

14. Do you suffer from hearing loss? When was the last time you had a hearing exam?

15. What do you do to relieve stress? How regularly do you engage in these activities?

16. Do you easily ask for help when in need? If not, write down the reasons and discuss them with your support group (family members, care givers, senior care center, friends, physician, etc.)

Which do you think is more important—physical health or mental health? Everyone is entitled to their opinion but I believe that mental health is far more vital. You might ask why. If you have a strong and healthy mind you can handle anything life throws at you, even physical ailments. I have seen this clearly in my patients suffering from chronic illness or cancer, or undergoing surgery. For instance, I have had patients with the same exact health condition undergoing knee or hip surgeries. Those who have gone into the surgery with a very stout psyche, a positive outlook, strong faith and deep family connections have had a much better surgical outcome and a much faster recovery. Those who were depressed, stressed, had a negative outlook, low or no spiritual connection, and weak family support had more complications and a much slower recovery.

A few years back I had a patient who had gone through a complex and complicated bladder surgery. Unfortunately, the surgery was unsuccessful and his bladder problem was worsened. After the surgery he was referred to my clinic by his primary care physician for a geriatric consult. From the moment he walked into my clinic with his daughter he was all smiles and laughs despite all the pains and discomforts he was experiencing. I enjoyed his visit so much and laughed as I had not in ages. I felt as though he was the one giving me all the right advice and cheering me rather than the other way around. During the follow-up visits we talked a lot about the bladder issues he had and about the surgery. And every time we laughed harder and longer than the last time he told me the story. He said once the surgery was over and he was in recovery the surgeon tried to explain to him, in a very grim face and his surgical cap in hand, that the surgery was not successful. And he said because of his language issues he did not understand a word of what the surgeon was telling him. He assumed the surgeon was telling him that all was now ok. He said he kept telling the surgeon "thank you doctor, thank you doctor" and kissed his hands over and over! The more he did this the more the surgeon bowed his head and stroked the patient's hands and he finally broke into tears. Again the patient thought the surgeon was so happy for him and that the tears were a sign of his joy. Following recovery he was brought to his room, the Foley Catheter was taken out, and he was asked to try to pee. He said, to his surprise, the pee was shooting high into the celling rather than into the urinal! His daughter finally told him about the outcome of the surgery and how he was not going to have a normal bladder moving forward. Instead of breaking down and crying he laughed and laughed and made fun of his language difficulties, the surgeon's face and disbelief, and his new bladder peeing against gravity. He refused to let his misfortune ruin his life and his dreams. And this is exactly what I am talking about in the above paragraph. With a strong and healthy mind you can take all the lemons life throws at you and turn them into lemonade.

So how can you develop, maintain or improve your mental health? While mental fitness and wellbeing partly depend on genetic makeup, life style choices and environmental factors play a major role on how you preserve or enhance your mental status as you age. We will discuss these key influencers in this chapter.

Physical Activity

As you will see in the next chapter it is imperative to stay physically active throughout life. Mild enjoyable exercises such as walking, swimming, gardening, dancing, yoga, or Tai Chi for 30 minutes a day improve/prevent memory loss and depression, and prevent dementia (including Alzheimer's).[1-5] A relaxing walk through a park (alone, with your friends, spouse, grandchildren or pet) or spending time in your garden planting herbs, flowers, vegetables, and fruit trees is all it takes.

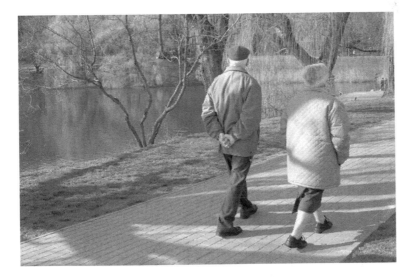

Most of these physical activities are free and widely available. You do not need to join an expensive gym full of state-of-the-art and intimidating sport gear. According to WR Hambrecht, in 2011 Americans spent $25.4 billion on professional sports (http://tinyurl.com/ajbdxoe)! Approximately, $2.6 billion per year are spent on gym memberships. While 15% of Americans have gym memberships (New York Times: http://tinyurl.com/o4yf3sv) only 8% actually show up at the gyms. And according to Ambient Insight (a market-research company) in 2009 Americans spent over $13 million on brain-fitness software and games (http://tinyurl.com/pyfxbbb). However, mild physical activities, free of charge, have the same effect on our mental fitness and health. In addition to its mental health benefits, regular exercise has many physical health benefits including

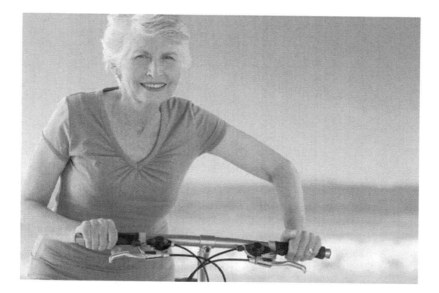

maintaining balance, preventing bone density and muscle mass loss, improving energy levels, decreasing blood pressure and cholesterol levels, and aiding in sustaining a healthy weight.

Get active and **have fun**. If it is not exciting, seems like a chore you keep putting off, or makes you procrastinate, and you imagine it as a torturous task each time you think of physical activity, then you are doing it wrong. While we emphasized moderation when it came to nutrition and diet in the previous chapter, mental fitness and health is all about stimulation and exhilaration.

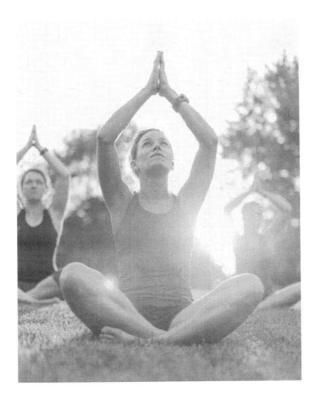

Note: In my practice, easy exercises like the ones suggested here have decreased the progression of dementia (including Alzheimer's) and lowered the rate of depression in my patients.

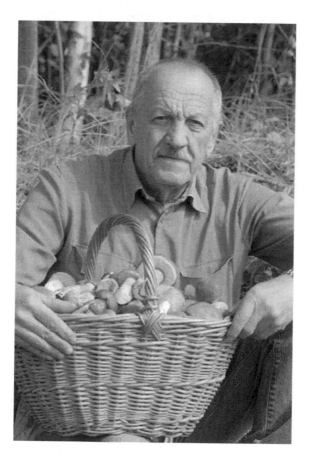

Nutrition

It is well established that healthy eating habits are essential for physical wellbeing. Nutritious foods strengthen our immune system and provide resistance to disease. Other benefits include better management of illnesses including chronic diseases and cancer as well as faster recuperation. Nutritious foods are also crucial for mental health, increasing mental acuteness, providing higher energy levels and emotional stability.

As stated in the previous chapter, try to eat organic foods free of chemicals, hormones, preservatives, herbicides and pesticides. Avoid drastic diets. Eat everything, in moderation, and stay away from canned, frozen and instant foods as much as possible. Limit your caffeine and alcohol intake. Caffeine interferes with sleep (which as you see below can interfere with memory) and also causes dehydration. Excessive alcohol consumption can result in memory loss and dehydration. Furthermore, alcohol can slow reaction time as well as cause dizziness, increasing the risk of falls and head injuries. Head injuries can result in both short- and long-term memory loss.

Smoking is a particularly harmful activity related to heart disease, hypertension, poor lung function, cancer, vascular (including cerebrovascular) disease and stroke. Stroke, which occurs when the blood supply (carrying oxygen and nutrients) to the brain is obstructed due to the blockage of a blood vessel to the brain or leakage of a blood vessel into the brain, causes memory loss. Cerebrovascular disease and stroke can result in cognitive decline and dementia. Furthermore, smoking causes memory impairment by reducing the amount of oxygen that gets to the brain.

What about the effect of vitamins and supplements in the prevention of dementia, including Alzheimer's, and in slowing the progression of cognitive impairment? Our cells utilize oxygen to metabolize nutrients. Therefore, oxygen has a vital role in our body for the production of energy. However, oxygen is highly reactive and can become part of damaging molecules called free radicals. These radicals can attack DNA, cell membranes, proteins and other macromolecules in our body, resulting in cell damage (such as in brain cell damage), aging and diseases. There have been a number of studies about the use of antioxidants (such as vitamins, minerals and supplements) including folate (a B vitamin), vitamins E, C, B6, B12, D and Beta Carotene for mental (and physical) health. The theory behind this is that antioxidants can deactivate free radicals and prevent damage to our DNA and cells. However, as we discussed in the Nutrition chapter, these results are inconclusive and highly debated. While a few small studies have shown the benefits of such antioxidants in prevention of dementia, large clinical studies have shown that vitamins and supplements are ineffective in treating and preventing Alzheimer's-type dementia and improving cognitive function.[6-9] And as we have discussed previously, taking extra levels of vitamins and supplements could be detrimental to our health. Therefore, unless your blood test results have indicated vitamin deficiencies, do not take over-the-counter supplements, minerals, vitamins and herbal remedies. You can get all the nutrients and vitamins your body requires from a healthy diet.

Staying Engaged (Social Engagement, Interaction and Support)

My wife's family lives in Canada and mine in Iran, while we live in California. So unfortunately, we do not have many family members around. Because of this, we make a point of socializing and interacting with our community as much as possible. We have an extended circle of friends, colleagues, and acquaintances we engage with quite often. We also do volunteer work, attend conferences, give talks, travel (for both business and pleasure), join new clubs (such as book, poetry, and movie clubs), take classes (such as wine, cooking and language classes), and find new hobbies quite often. You might ask why? Studies have shown that people who stay socially engaged with their family, friends, community and environment and have an active and adaptive lifestyle have a much better mental health. They are less depressed, maintain cognitive functions until much later in life, take much longer to show symptoms of dementia (including Alzheimer's disease), and have a lower risk of disability and mortality.[10-15] It is all about having endeavors you are enthusiastic about in life and sharing them with people who can enjoy them as much as you do.

A year ago I came across a highly educated patient in my clinic. She lived with her husband. They were both recently retired and since giving up work had maintained a very monotonous lifestyle. She was severely depressed and withdrawn. She would not eat, did not enjoy life as she once had and was becoming very frail. During one of her visits to my office, I asked her if she had any hobbies. She looked at me puzzled. I asked her if she liked traveling, bicycling, swimming, painting, or enjoyed any other social activity. She said she always wanted to try photography. I asked her to take a few pictures of things she found interesting in her surroundings and perhaps share them with me and her friends. She did. She and her husband picked up a camera and took such spectacular pictures of the wilderness as well as their stunning backyard and everything that was happening in it. They took pictures of birds, trees, rabbits, and flowers. With her permission, I have included one of these pictures that she gave us for the birth of our son with a letter she enclosed in this book. Once she started her new hobby, she began to recover from her depression, started eating again and showed great improvement in her general health. She is full of energy these days, and I can't tell you how enthusiastic I am seeing the new pictures she shares with me during each visit. She has found a new meaning for life and discovered something to be passionate about, something to look forward to. It also provided a means for her to share her joy with others, even her doctor, and interact with the world outside her door.

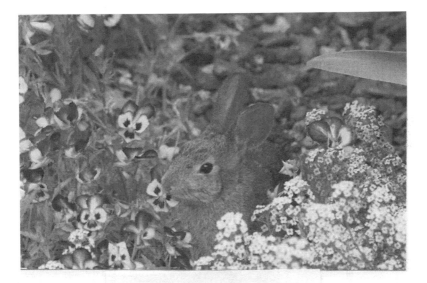

Dear Hope and Mehrdad,

Thank you so much for sending photos of Sam. As of May 1st we have had a small rabbit in our garden and we have taken many pictures of it. It was very tiny at first and we are watching it grow and change. It is beginning to eat our flowers now, not just grass and weeds. Three days ago I took this picture in the early morning. When ▓▓ printed it for my book, I immediately thought, "Sam should have one, too."

With our best wishes,

As I mentioned to you, in 2013 we had the biggest miracle of our life—our son was born. When I found out that we were going to have a baby I started sharing the news with many of my patients and kept them in the loop with the progress, from what we were expecting to when the due date was, to the name we picked out, and all the other information expecting parents are highly excited about. To my amusement, most of my patients became highly engaged in the process. They showered us with gifts they had hand made for us (paintings, socks, hats, blankets, etc.), valuable advice, and affection. We loved it since with no family around we needed all the precious support we could get. It was amazing what revelations I saw in my patients. I started seeing less depression among them. It was remarkable how they remembered all the details I had given them! They also became more open and sharing with me, the nurses, and their caregivers. During each visit, the conversations started tilting more toward the baby rather than the ailments they had! As a matter of fact they would state that the main reason they would now make appointments was to bring us gifts, inquire about the baby's health, see the newest baby pictures, give us advice on how to properly take care of him, and if possible, to see him. When I asked about their health and medical conditions, the majority reported much better mental and physical health. We all want to have a reason to feel excited, to love and be loved, to feel needed and alive. We can only do this by staying engaged with the society around us.

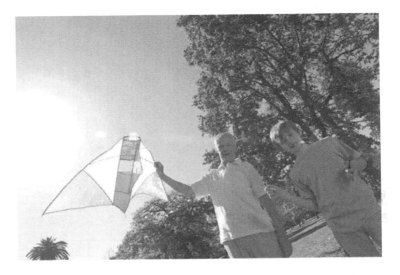

One of the problems with our society is that as people get older they become less engaged with the younger generation. They retire to the solitude of their homes. Their children and grandchildren move away or have busy lives with almost no time to spare. Slowly, they become isolated from the world and depression begins to set in. Or perhaps they retire in senior care facilities where they are only exposed to people who are within the same age bracket and have similar physical and mental ailments as themselves! Just like them they have lost spouses, family members, friends, and feel abandoned and lonely. The solution these facilities offer to help with depression is to encourage seniors to interact with one another (such as eat together, play games, listen to music, watch TV, etc.). However, these interactions are again between people with similar mental and health status, and the results can be dismal. If this sounds familiar, my advice is to find at least one activity (such as tutoring, volunteering, or teaching) that allows you to interact with the younger generation. It is amazing how much you can enjoy their company. They are like a breath of fresh air—full of life, energy, new ideas, motivation and aspiration. Ever since I became a teacher and a father there is not a single day that has passed without me learning a new skill, mastering a new subject and feeling more alive than ever. And what you can teach them from a lifetime of experiences is invaluable.

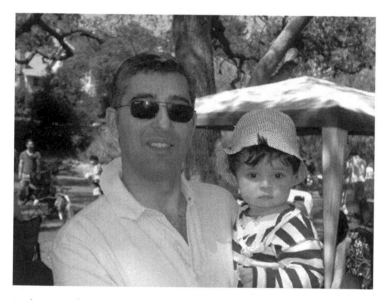

A picture of Dr. Ayati with his son Sam

It is in human nature to want to stay physically, emotionally and financially independent as much as possible throughout life. However, as we age we might unavoidably need support and help from our community. Reluctance to ask for help may stem from the fear of losing our independence, integrity and sense of worth. It might be frightening and painful to see that we are losing the ability to care for ourselves. However, rest assured that there is no shame in asking for help that you really need, regardless of your age. Rather, it's a sign of strength. You can ask your neighbors, friends, family members, doctors or other care providers, members of your church/synagogue/mosque/temple/ senior center for support and still live a proud, independent and fulfilling life. You will be amazed at how eager people are to help if only you ask them. And if you are still hesitant in asking for support ponder on this: If the tables were turned and someone needed your help, what would be your advice to them?

In short, focus on activities that make you happy. Surround yourself with people of all ages. Interact with, support and get support from your community.

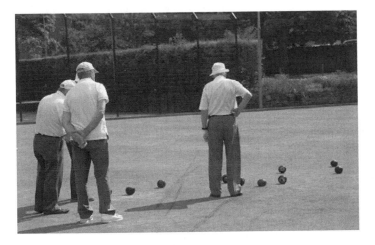

Spirituality

A while ago I was doing a routine medical round in one of the nursing homes I attend. I came across two patients in the hallway who were in a heated discussion over spirituality and its benefits. One of them strongly believed in the power of spirituality while the other considered it a waste of time. The believer said, "Imagine being stranded, all alone, in a broken boat, in the middle of a storm somewhere in the Atlantic Ocean. There is very little hope in surviving. What would be your first reaction and what would be the first thought that comes across your mind?" The other patient thought for a while and said, "Well, needless to say that there is nothing to be done. I would be scared to death and just think this is the end." The believer said, "That is why I want to believe in a higher force. Call it God, nature, energy, aliens, or whatever name you choose. First of all, it allows me to have hope to survive, and therefore I pray instead of focusing on the misfortune. Second, I don't feel alone since this higher being is with me throughout my journey-whatever it might be. And, it gives me a peace of mind in case I conclude that I would not survive. It gives me a sense of harmony and serenity to know that my life had a purpose, that it was not all for nothing and that someone or another journey is awaiting me on the other side. This would make the tragedy less scary, and it would be easier to surrender." The other patient pondered on this and said, "It would certainly be a lot more scary and final for me."

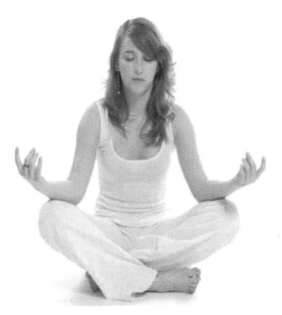

People turn toward spirituality or organized religion for many reasons. Among them are to search for a meaning or purpose in life, to cope with difficult situations such as illness, stress or loss of loved ones, for peace, comfort, connectedness, altruism, or out of gratefulness. Studies have shown a positive relationship between spirituality and happiness, physical and mental health, faster recovery from illness, slower progression of Alzheimer's, greater social support, and a higher quality of life.[16-22] They also indicate that spirituality decreases anxiety, depression, low self-esteem, fear, stress and loneliness, and reduces the likelihood of drug and alcohol abuse. Spirituality can bring hope, peace, forgiveness, positive emotions, and a feeling of well-being. Whatever the reason, set aside some time to meditate, to connect with nature and perhaps the universe, or just focus on yourself through breathing exercises or on living healthier. You can also focus on others through volunteering and the act of giving.

Mind and Intellectual Stimulation

My wife once told me the most hilarious story about when her mom was in her late thirties. During this time my wife was attending university. On numerous occasions she had clearly mentioned to her mother that she was going to get home late at night since she had finals and needed to study at the library. However, during those nights her mom would be wondering where she had been and was worried sick. On one occasion her mom even called the police and reported her missing. I would like to remind you that during those days there were no cell phones. My wife finally got worried about her mom's mental status and went to her university's library in search of answers. Again, let me remind you that there was no internet during those days either and people actually went to libraries to do research. She diagnosed her mom with Alzheimer's based on articles she read in their health library and consequently made an appointment for her mom with a very renowned neurologist. During the visit the very young and handsome doctor (as my wife referred to him) was utterly puzzled about the purpose of their visit. My wife explained that her mom was becoming very forgetful and that she thought her mom had Alzheimer's disease. The doctor chuckled and told my wife not to waste his precious time, which could be spent on seeing real patients. My wife became very offended and asked for an explanation. The doctor told my wife that her mom was very healthy and based on the questionnaire she answered had no dementia. The reason why she was becoming forgetful was that she was experiencing some degree of stress (she was in the process of a divorce) in her life and as a result was easily distracted. Furthermore, as she was no longer in her twenties when our cognitive abilities reach their peak versus in our thirties when they start a shallow decline, some degree of forgetfulness was considered normal. The only recommendation he had was for her mom to pick up the phone book and memorize numbers to keep her mind active and her memory sharp.

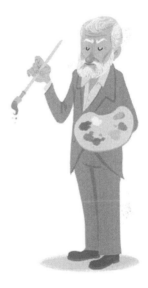

Studies have indicated that our ability to preserve or improve our mental status as we age depends largely on our life style choices. For instance, our level of education, occupation, linguistic ability, and leisure pursuits are all factors that affect our ability to grow intellectually, and therefore our mental health.[10, 23-26] Simply picking up a phone book and memorizing numbers or doing crosswords would not do it.[27] What is of utmost importance is our ability to engage in new stimulating activities that are outside of our comfort zone. Hence, find a variety of novel and exciting activities you always wanted to try and never had time to before. Learn new fun skills such as painting, playing an instrument, ballroom dancing, poker, sculpturing, etc. Traveling, dating, playing a new sport, learning a foreign language, or wild mushroom picking are all challenging activities, which can help us build brain capacity. However, the two key factors are first to choose **a new activity** (the task should never become routine or easy) and second **to enjoy it**. If you do not enjoy it, there is no benefit in it. Do not make this into another chore you have to do. Instead turn it into a set of experiences you have always dreamed about.

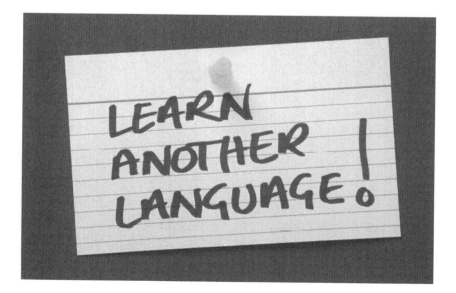

Note: As we age some of our mental abilities such as wisdom, social skills, emotional intelligence, and self-control actually improve; these are great traits to share with others. Therefore, we have many positive things to look forward to as we age.

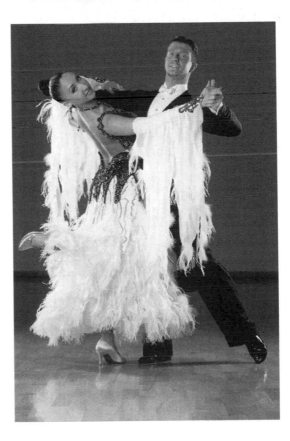

Stress Reduction

In our society productivity is highly valued. It is the ruling law of the land. Unfortunately, our sense of self-worth may become based on our rate of productivity. We are actively encouraged to multitask and be highly efficient, smart, resourceful, and perfectionists. In order to accomplish all this we need to keep running in high gear 24/7 (if you don't believe me, see how many times you checked your emails today). Financial hardship, demanding family life, exhausting work schedules and commutes, and lack of sleep are among the factors that lead to stress. Long term exposure to stress has adverse health consequences. It can result in high blood pressure, suppress our immune system, increase the risk of stroke and heart attack, and speed up the aging process. It can also lead to anxiety and depression. It is well established that emotional problems such as stress, anxiety and depression are linked to six of the leading causes of death, namely heart, lung and liver diseases, cancer, accidents, and suicide.

These emotional problems can lead to compulsive behaviors such as overeating or anorexia, and substance abuse with alcohol, tobacco, or drugs. They cause sleep disruption, which can lead to fatigue and interfere with the ability to consolidate and retrieve information. They can affect our level of concentration (by overstimulation or distraction), attention and focus, and even result in memory loss.

Life is not a race. We do not have to be perfect and live in a cookie cutter society. We do not have to keep up appearances and have nothing to prove to anyone including ourselves. We do not need to conform to what the media and our society expect of us. We are on a journey, and each one of us individually needs to focus on how to live a happy, fulfilling, and meaningful life. We are entitled to stop many times along the way and smell the roses. Try to steer yourself away from stress, anxiety and depression.

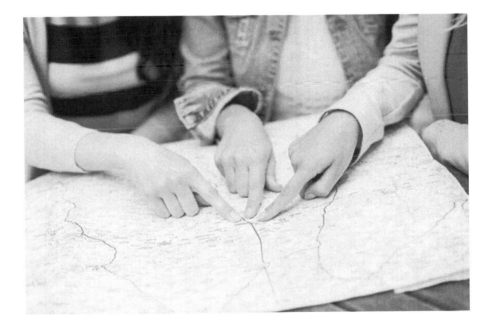

Relaxation techniques such as meditation to increase your inner awareness, stillness and balance, massage, aromatherapy and exercise, such as yoga, deep breathing, Tai Chi, etc. are very helpful stress reducers. Joining support groups, talking to trusted friends and family members, reducing your caffeine intake (overuse of caffeine interferes with sleep and sleep deprivation results in memory loss), and simply taking time off from everyday life routines (traffic jams, cell phones and computers) are among the many ways one can also get stress relief.

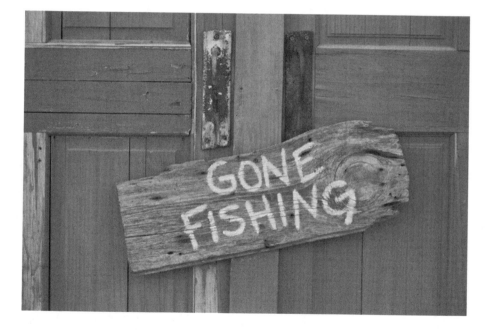

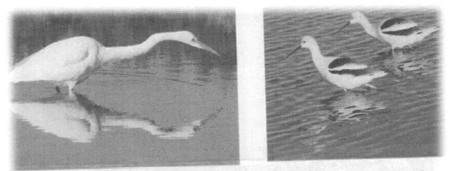

Great Egret   San Francisco Bayshore   Avocets

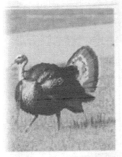
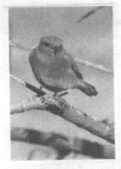
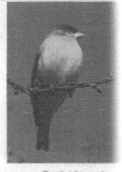

Wild Turkey   Bluebird   Goldfinch

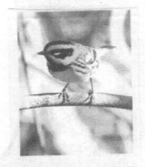

Townsend's Warbler

One of my patients chose bird watching as a way of relaxation

65

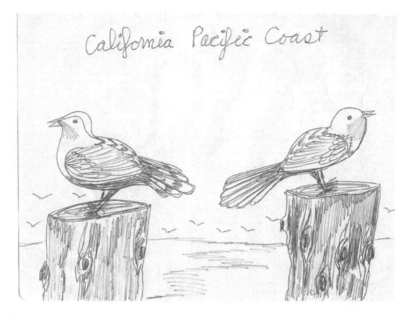

A patient of mine chose bird drawing as a way of relaxation

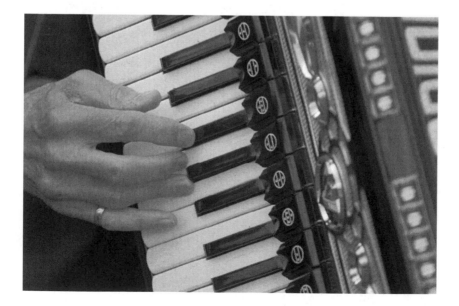

I have talked about my father before. He is currently in his early eighties and still works as an ophthalmologist. At least twice a month he drives for miles on narrow winding roads from the capital Tehran to the Caspian Sea in the north where my parents own a chalet. He lives a very healthy, happy and engaged life. He eats all he wishes, which includes lots of carbohydrates (in the form of rice, breads, and pastries) and fats (in the form of meats, nuts and eggs). He has never been on any sort of diet or medication. His memory seems as sharp as it was in his twenties. Do you know what his secret is? He

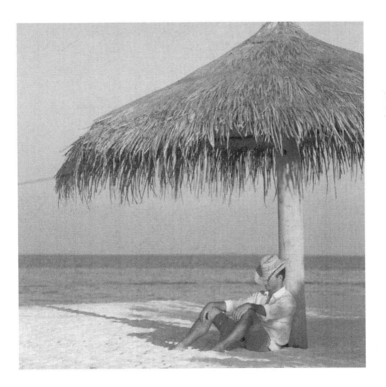

lives a very relaxed and joyful life. He never lets any issue bother him. He never envies anyone and never holds a grudge. And he **never** skips his naps. In Iran, just as in Spain, Turkey, Greece, and Italy, people take siestas. These are short, up to two hours, naps in the middle of the day. They have been shown to decrease stress, reduce heart attack and coronary mortality (by 37%), and enhance information processing, performance, memory and learning.[28-30] It is interesting that most research done on the benefit of naps was performed in the US. However in America, many consider napping an act of laziness and a sign of poor productivity! Take your naps if you can and don't feel guilty about it. Medical science is on your side.

Medication

The elderly take far too many prescription drugs as well as over-the-counter (OTC) medications and supplements. You will see from the Overmedication chapter that as we age we become more sensitive to medications and their side effects. These medications can cross-react and severely affect our physical and mental health. The problem becomes life threatening if on top of that we drink alcohol. In addition to causing (often irreversible) physiological damages, these medications can increase risk of falls, accidents, and injuries.

Let's consider a few examples of medications interfering with your mental health in this chapter. Anti-anxiety, anti-insomnia, antidepressants, anti-psychotics, antihistamines, as well as muscle relaxants, tranquilizers and pain medications can all have side effects of excessive sleepiness and grogginess. They can cause confusion, disorientation, hallucinations, seizures and delirium, as well as problems with attention and concentration. They may even trigger memory loss. Anticancer medications, anti-inflammatory drugs and progesterone are known to be associated with depression. Always check with your physician before taking any prescription or even OTC medications.

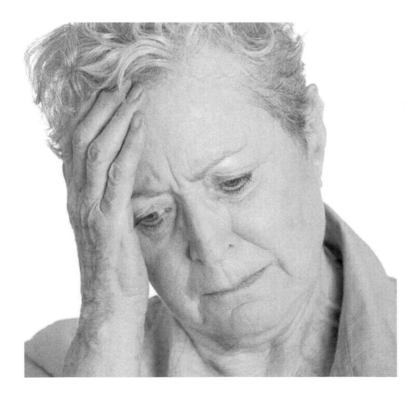

Physical Health

You have probably heard from your physicians on the subject of hypertension (high blood pressure) and hypercholesterolemia (high cholesterol), warning you that both can have dire effects on your mental and physical health. Let's discuss these two subjects here.

For many years now researchers have been trying unsuccessfully to find a cure for Alzheimer's and vascular dementia. Vascular dementia is caused when the blood flow to the brain is blocked or reduced as a result of stroke(s) and/or small vessel disease (narrowed or damaged blood vessels). Blockage can be caused by blood clots, by plaque build-up on the inside of artery walls or by aneurysm (when a section of an artery wall forms an outward balloon and bursts). If oxygen and nutrients don't reach the brain cells, they die, resulting in permanent brain damage. Depending on the area of the brain involved, the damages could include memory loss, and/or problems with learning, reasoning, judgment, and planning. Scientists have found that risk factors for vascular dementia include hypertension, hypercholesterolemia, diabetes, lupus, cerebrovascular and cardiovascular disease, smoking, temporal arteritis, and age. Multiple trials were set up to see if antihypertensive medications (medications that lower blood pressure) could prevent dementia. Unfortunately, they found that lowering blood pressure did not prevent the development of dementia or cognitive impairment in hypertensive patients or in patients suffering from cardiovascular disease or diabetes.[31, 32]

It is still reasonable to treat hypertension because of the many health benefits of doing so. **However, one very important note of caution is that what is considered a normal blood pressure in a young adult is different from that in the elderly.** In young adults a healthy blood pressure is 120 (systolic) over 80 (diastolic) mmHg. However, as per most academic geriatric societies, a systolic blood pressure between 135-140 mmHg and a diastolic blood pressure between 70-90 mmHg is considered normal for the elderly. Reducing the blood pressure to lower than these levels and thus over-treating blood pressure in the geriatric population is of great concern. There are two reasons for this. As we age, we require a higher blood perfusion to our brain in order to restore our cognition. If our blood pressure drops below the range recommended above, the blood perfusion to our brain drops, putting us at a higher risk of confusion and memory loss. Another reason is that orthostatic hypotension (also called a dizzy spell) is more prevalent among the elderly. Orthostatic hypotension occurs when there is a sudden drop in a person's blood pressure when standing up, moving or stretching. This is a serious condition occurring in 20% of the elderly and can result in acute hospitalization. Symptoms include dizziness, nausea, headache, euphoria, loss of hearing, blurred vision, seizure, and fainting. Therefore, make sure to discuss this with your physician before taking antihypertensive medications or OTC supplements or herbal remedies.

What about cholesterol and its effect on dementia? Most people know that high blood cholesterol is a risk factor for heart disease, but it is a risk factor for dementia as well. Yet just as we saw in the case of antihypertensive medications, researchers have not been able to show that cholesterol lowering medications can prevent cognitive decline or dementia in the elderly.[33] My recommendation to my patients is to lower their cholesterol through the life style changes we have been discussing so far. They should eat healthy diets, exercise moderately, and lower their stress levels. If they are then unable to lower their cholesterol level despite a healthy life style (due to genetic factors, for example), then I prescribe cholesterol lowering medications for them. **However, I also want to mention that over-treating high cholesterol is as problematic as over-treating high blood pressure in the elderly.** Often I have seen patients on cholesterol lowering medication even though their LDL (bad cholesterol) is well within the normal range. Normal LDL is different in each individual and is dependent on risk factors such as history of stroke, heart disease, diabetes, smoking, etc. If their risk of forming blood clots is high, they could be at a higher risk of stroke and vascular disease and their normal level of LDL should be lower than an individual with no risk factors. Your physician can determine the risk factors for you as an individual.

Note: It is worth mentioning that when you get your cholesterol results from laboratories they come with limit numbers (called the reference interval), which are considered "normal". Anything outside of that range is considered high or low and shows up with an asterisk or flag next to your results. You need to discuss this with your physician and let him or her determine your healthy level of cholesterol based on your known risk factors.

Another medical condition having a direct effect on your cognition and memory is hearing loss. The hearing-impaired are more likely to experience cognitive and memory problems than those with normal hearing. Elderly who have hearing problems experience cognitive decline 30 to 40 percent faster than those with normal hearing.[34] What are the possible explanations for this? MRI results in the people experiencing hearing loss show activation of prefrontal cortex (an area normally focused on memory) to help auditory processing. The brain is therefore reallocating resources to help with hearing at the expense of cognition. Furthermore, as we learned, one of the major risk factors for dementia is social isolation. People who have hearing loss are more prone to social isolation. If you do experience hearing loss, you are not alone. In America, more than 26 million people over the age of 50 suffer from it. It is vital to seek help and there are many ways to restore your hearing (such as by using a hearing aid or by cochlear implant). Make an appointment with your physician to resolve this issue as soon as possible.

Take Home Message

In order to maintain and improve your mental health and cognitive functions you need to do the following:

- Eat a healthy diet
- Stay socially engaged
- Reduce your stress level
- Participate in fun physical exercises
- Invigorate your mind with enjoyable activities
- Seek support whenever needed
- Engage in preventative care by visiting your physician routinely

ACTION PLAN

1. Make a list of your favorite hobbies and make a plan to engage in them

2. Make a list of new activities you would like to try and make a plan to engage in them

3. Make an appointment with your doctor to check your hearing

4. Make a list of all the people in your support system and make sure you meet with them on a regular basis

5. Make a list of activities you engage in to relieve stress

6. Try to take a nap (even if it is on the weekend) and see how you feel after you nap

REFERENCES

1. The association between physical activity and dementia in an elderly population: the Rotterdam Study. de Bruijn RF, Schrijvers EM, de Groot KA, Witteman JC, Hofman A, Franco OH, Koudstaal PJ, Ikram MA, Eur J Epidemiol. 2013;28(3):277-83.

2. Watermemories: a swimming club for adults with dementia. Neville C, Clifton K, Henwood T, Beattie E, McKenzie MA, J Gerontol Nurs. 2013 Feb;39(2):21-5.

3. The Mental Activity and eXercise (MAX) trial: a randomized controlled trial to enhance cognitive function in older adults. Barnes DE, Santos-Modesitt W, Poelke G, Kramer AF, Castro C, Middleton LE, Yaffe K, JAMA Intern Med. 2013;173(9):797-804.

4. Mood alteration with swimming-swimmers really do "feel better". Berger BG, Owen DR, Psychosom Med. 1983;45(5):425-33.

5. Physical activity and common mental disorders. Harvey SB, Hotopf M, Overland S, Mykletun A, Br J Psychiatry. 2010;197(5):357-64.

6. A randomized trial of vitamin E supplementation and cognitive function in women. Kang JH, Cook N, Manson J, Buring JE, Grodstein F, Arch Intern Med. 2006;166(22):2462.

7. Impact of antioxidants, zinc, and copper on cognition in the elderly: a randomized, controlled trial. Yaffe K, Clemons TE, McBee WL, Lindblad AS, Age-Related Eye Disease Study Research Group, Neurology. 2004;63(9):1705.

8. Vitamin E and donepezil for the treatment of mild cognitive impairment. Petersen RC, Thomas RG, Grundman M, Bennett D, Doody R, Ferris S, Galasko D, Jin S, Kaye J, Levey A, Pfeiffer E, Sano M, van Dyck CH, Thal LJ, Alzheimer's Disease Cooperative Study Group, N Engl J Med. 2005;352(23):2379.

9. Antioxidants and prevention of cognitive decline: does duration of use matter? Yaffe Arch, Intern Med. 2007;167(20):2167.

10. An integrated and socially integrated lifestyle in late life might protect against dementia. Fratiglioni L, Paillard-Borg S, and Winblad B, Lancet Neurol. 2004; 3:343.

11. Late-life engagement in social and leisure activities is associated with a decreased risk of dementia: a longitudinal study from the Kungsholmen project. Wang HX, Karp A, Winblad B, Fratiglioni L, Am J Epidemiol. 2002;155(12):1081-7.

12. Social engagement and health outcomes among older people: introduction to a special section. Bath PA, Deeg D, Eur J Ageing. 2005;2: 24–30.

13. Low level social engagement as a precursor of mortality among people in later life. Bennett KM, Age Ageing. 2002;31: 165–168.

14. Social engagement and disability in a community population of older adults: the New Haven EPESE. Mendes de Leon CF, Glass TA, Berkman LF, Am J Epidemiol. 2003; 157: 633–642.

15. Social activity and improvement in depressive symptoms in older people: a prospective community cohort study. Isaac V, Stewart R, Artero S, Ancelin ML, Ritchie K, Am J Geriatr Psychiatry. 2009; 17: 688–696.

16. "Religious attendance and cognitive functioning among older Mexican Americans". Hill TD, Burdette AM, Angel JL, and Angel RJ, Journals of Gerontology. 2006; B, vol. 61, no. 1, pp. P3–P9.

17. Cognitive decline in Alzheimer's disease. Impact of spirituality, religiosity, and QOL. Kaufman Y, Anaki D, Binns M, Freedman M, Neurology. 2007;68:1509-1514.

18. An increase in religiousness/spirituality occurs after HIV diagnosis and predicts slower disease progression over 4 years in people with HIV. Ironson G, Stuetzle R, Fletcher MA, J Gen Intern Med. 2006;21 Suppl 5:S62-8.

19. The affective profiles in the USA: happiness, depression, life satisfaction, and happiness-increasing strategies. Schütz E, Sailer U, Al Nima A, Rosenberg P, Andersson Arntén AC, Archer T, Garcia D, PeerJ. 2013;1:e156.

20. Mental disorders, religion and spirituality 1990 to 2010: a systematic evidence-based review. Bonelli RM, Koenig HG, J Relig Health. 2013;52(2):657-73.

21. Nursing home care: exploring the role of religiousness in the mental health, quality of life and stress of formal caregivers. Lucchetti G, Lucchetti AL, Oliveira GR, Crispim D, Pires SL, Gorzoni ML, Panicio CR, Koenig HG, J Psychiatr Ment Health Nurs. 2013 May 23.

22. The effects of a spiritual learning program on improving spiritual health and clinical practice stress among nursing students. Hsiao YC, Chiang HY, Lee HC, Chen SH, J Nurs Res. 2012;20(4):281-90.

23. Brain-stimulating habits linked to lower Alzheimer's protein levels. Research shows that a lifetime of mentally challenging activities may help delay dementia. Duke Med Health News. 2012;18(4):3.

24. Effectiveness of cognitive training for Chinese elderly in Hong Kong. Kwok T, Wong A, Chan G, Shiu YY, Lam KC, Young D, Ho DW, Ho F, Clin Interv Aging. 2013;8:213-9.

25. Cognitive change and the APOE epsilon 4 allele. Deary IJ, Whiteman MC, Pattie A, Starr JM, Hayward C, Wright AF, Carothers A, Whalley LJ, Nature. 2002; 418, 932.

26. Remembering numbers in old age: Mnemonic training versus self-generated strategy training. Derwinger, A, Neely, AS, Persson M, Hill RD, Backman L, Aging Neuropsychol C. 2003;10(3), 202-214.

27. Predictors of crossword puzzle proficiency and moderators of age-cognition relations. Hambrick, DZ, Salthouse, TA, Meinz EJ, Journal of Experimental Psychology: General. 1999;128, 131-164.

28. Siesta in healthy adults and coronary mortality in the general population. Naska A, Oikonomou E, Trichopoulou A, Psaltopoulou T, Trichopoulos D, Archives of Internal Medicine. 2007; 167, 296-301.

29. Sleep-dependent learning: a nap is as good as a night. Mednick S, Nakayama K, Stickgold R, Nat Neurosci. 2003;6(7):697-8.

30. The restorative effect of naps on perceptual deterioration. Mednick SC, Nakayama K, Cantero JL, Atienza M, Levin AA, Pathak N, Stickgold R, Nat Neurosci. 2002;5(7):677-81.

31. Blood pressure lowering in patients without prior cerebrovascular disease for prevention of cognitive impairment and dementia. McGuinness B, Todd S, Passmore P, Bullock R, Cochrane Database Syst Rev. 2009;(4):CD004034.

32. Renin-angiotensin system blockade and cognitive function in patients at high risk of cardiovascular disease: analysis of data from the ONTARGET and TRANSCEND studies. Anderson C, Teo K, Gao P, Arima H, Dans A, Unger T, Commerford P, Dyal L, Schumacher H, Pogue J, Paolasso E, Holwerda N, Chazova I, Binbrek A, Young J, Yusuf S; ONTARGET and TRANSCEND Investigators, Lancet Neurol. 2011;10(1):43-53.

33. Statins for prevention of dementia, McGuinness B, Craig D, Bullock R, Passamore P, Cochrane Database Syst Rev.2009.

34. Hearing loss could be linked to dementia. Treat age-related hearing loss to help prevent dementia. Duke Med Health News. 2013;19(5):1-2.

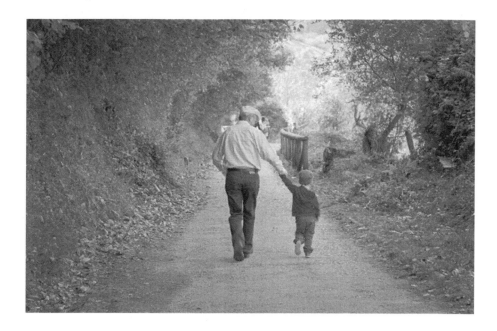

Chapter 3

Frailty

Questions to Ask Yourself

1. Do you experience any of the following symptoms?
   - Lack of energy
   - Overtiredness
   - Feebleness
   - Lack of strength
   - Inability to do any tasks
   - Dizziness
   - Loss of balance
   - Recent history of falls
   - Lack of appetite

2. Do you suffer from any chronic illness, cancer or mental illness?

3. Have you been diagnosed with osteoporosis? Has your doctor determined the cause and addressed it?

4. What type of exercises do you do and how many times a week? Have these exercises helped you improve your strength, stamina, balance, and appetite?

5. Are you depressed? Do you see a doctor for your depression regularly? Ask your doctor to determine the underlying cause of your depression and a plan for action. If you are taking anti-depressants have they helped you or are they resulting in further loss of appetite, immobility, confusion and delirium?

Many patients walk in to my clinic complaining about a lack of energy, overtiredness, feebleness, a lack of strength, inability, dizziness, loss of balance, a recent history of falls, and a lack of appetite. What they suffer from is called *frailty*. They ask me for a quick fix—perhaps a pill, an injection of vitamin B, a prescription for iron, or a recommendation for over the counter vitamins and supplements. My answer to them is that there is no magic pill. Vitamins and supplements, as previously discussed in the Nutrition chapter, are not the answer.

Frailty is defined as a progressive deterioration of multiple body systems resulting in physical and functional decline. It is characterized as a drop in the body's energy production and utilization as well as a deterioration of its repair systems. Frailty is the result of the natural aging process (physiological impairments), medical conditions (such as chronic diseases, cancer and infectious diseases) and environmental factors (such as lifestyle choices). It can occur at any age but is much more prevalent in the elderly. It is marked by an increased susceptibility to illness, falls, disability, immobility, depression, cognitive impairment, institutionalization, and death. In clinical terms, a person is diagnosed with frailty if they have three or more of the following factors: Unintended weight loss of more than 5% of body weight in one year, exhaustion, weakness, low levels of physical activity, and physical and mental slowness.[1-5] It is therefore imperative to prevent frailty and reverse its process or halt its progression immediately. The good news is that this can often be accomplished. In this chapter we will review the risk factors playing major roles in frailty as well as methods of prevention and treatment.

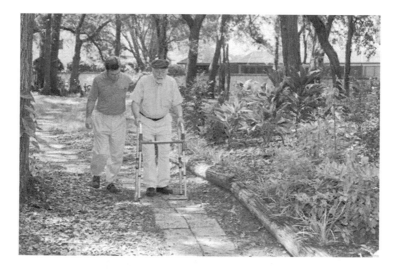

Loss of Appetite

As mentioned in the Nutrition chapter, loss of appetite is inevitable as we age. We are physically less active. Our metabolism decreases. We lose our taste buds, our sense of smell declines and we are more prone to dental problems. Our body undergoes hormonal changes, which lead to earlier and more pronounced satiety with small meals. We also have reduced gastric motility. Furthermore, chronic diseases, cancer, hormone (such as testosterone) deficiency, psychological disorders (such as depression & anxiety) and medications can also result in loss of appetite. Elderly who suffer from eating problems are more subject to malnutrition and as a consequence weight loss, fatigue, weakness, and ultimately frailty.[6,7] It is therefore vital to maintain a healthy balanced diet by eating nutritious foods. For more information about nutrition and how to prevent weight loss refer to Chapter I of this book.

Loss of Muscle Mass (Sarcopenia)

As we grow older we eventually lose about 40 percent of our muscle tissue. It is replaced by fat. The reason for this loss is that people over the age of 65 build muscles less efficiently compared to younger people. And the mechanism that prevents muscle breakdown works less effectively in the elderly. Therefore, we can't build and repair muscles as quickly as we did in our younger years. This could be explained by the fact that blood flow carrying nutrients and hormones necessary for building and repairing muscles is lower in the older people. Other factors such as a decrease in the level of physical activity, hormone (testosterone and growth hormone) deficiencies, medications (corticosteroids prescribed for asthma or inflammatory conditions such as rheumatoid arthritis and lupus), and medical issues (such as cancer or nerve diseases) can further accelerate this process. A decrease in muscle mass can lead to weakness, falls, pain, chronic inflammation, and immobility, in turn leading to frailty.[8] This loss of muscle mass, or sarcopenia, also results in loss of immune function as well as brain cell death and impairment of cognition and memory.[9, 10]

The good news is that sarcopenia is preventable and, if detected early, reversible. Nutrition and exercise are the two key factors. A diet rich in high quality proteins is a must. Proteins (also called amino acids) are the building blocks of muscles. Therefore, if you're an omnivore, make sure to include meat, eggs and dairy in your daily diet. Beans, legumes, grains and nuts are also a good source of proteins. However, due to their high fiber content their digestion becomes harder as we age. Meat has no fiber and is thus more easily digested. If you follow a vegetarian or vegan diet you will need to eat a combination of plant proteins (for example, brown rice and black beans, hummus and whole wheat pita, whole wheat toast with peanut butter) over the course of a day in order to get all the proteins your body requires (for more information refer to the following handout from Iowa State University: http://tinyurl.com/pogsr6c).

In order to maintain or build your muscles it is also crucial to perform muscle strengthening exercises. Besides making you stronger, these exercises improve your bone density and prevent osteoporosis (see below). They also enhance your coordination, flexibility, mobility, range of motion and balance and help reduce the symptoms of chronic diseases such as arthritis, diabetes, pulmonary and cardiovascular disease, stroke, back pain, depression and obesity.[11] Additionally, strength training exercises improve sleep quality by helping us fall asleep faster, sleep more deeply, awaken less often, and sleep longer. As we learned in the previous chapter, you need good quality sleep to improve your memory. And remember that when you exercise, you increase your level of activity, you take in more calories, and you stimulate your appetite.

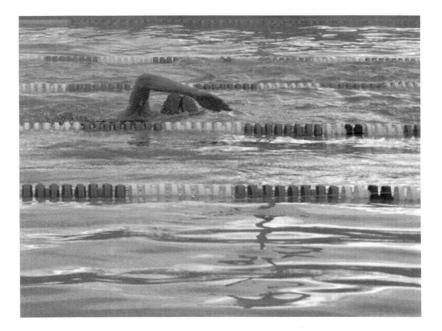

We discussed aerobic exercises such as walking, swimming, gardening, dancing, biking, or pushing a lawn mower in the Mental Health chapter. They increase our fitness and endurance. Strength (or resistance) training exercises, on the other hand, are the ones that make our muscles strong and increase our muscle mass and bone density. They also improve our tolerance and walking speed. These exercises involve lifting weights and working with resistance bands. Similarly to aerobic activities, resistance exercises require little time and minimal equipment. For instance, lifting weights could be accomplished by lifting pans, pots or books around the house. Therefore, there is no need to join gyms or purchase expensive gear.

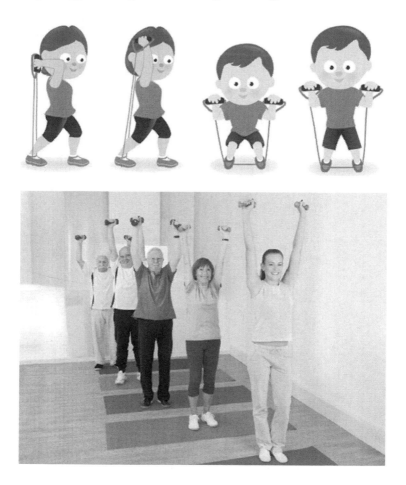

The American College of Sports Medicine (ACSM) and The American Heart Association (AHA) have come up with a great guideline for workouts that include both muscle strengthening and endurance (aerobic) exercises.[12] I have been using this guideline on my patients with great results to counteract weakness and frailty and for promoting and maintaining health. According to this guideline, older adults need to perform mild aerobic exercises (like the ones mentioned above) five days a week for a minimum of 30 minutes and perform strength training (strenuous) exercises at least twice per week.

Strenuous exercises should engage all your major muscles (like the ones in your arms, shoulders, legs, hips, back, chest and abdomen area). Examples include lifting weights, working with resistance bands, calisthenics, and using body weight for resistance in exercises such as push-ups, pull ups and sit ups. Climbing stairs is also very beneficial if you do not suffer from knee or hip arthritis. You should do 8-10 such exercises at least twice per week and each exercise should be repeated 8-12 times. The key point here is to start with light weights as well as low strength resistance bands and build strength before moving to heavier ones. Don't lift a 20 pound weight on the first day and harm yourself. Remember that this is not a race but a joyful endeavor that promotes health and fitness. It can only be accomplished by patience.

Note: If you suffer from a chronic disease (cardiovascular disease, arthritis, diabetes, etc.), it is vital to start your exercise programs under the care of your physician. Your doctor can tell you about the types and amounts of physical activity that are appropriate for you and refer you to the right physical therapist. Remember that moderation is the theme throughout this book. Do not attempt to lift heavy weights or exercise obsessively. It can have adverse effects on your health.

Bone Loss (Osteoporosis)

Osteoporosis is an age-related bone disease in which you lose your bone mass. Your bones become weak, porous, brittle, and prone to fracture, especially in the areas of the hip, spine and wrist. Other causes such as hormone deficiencies (estrogen in women, testosterone in men, parathyroid hormone and growth hormone), medications (such as corticosteroids), low intake of calcium and vitamin D, poor life style choices (such as a sedentary lifestyle, smoking, and high alcohol consumption), and medical conditions (such as paralysis, thyroid problems, genetic diseases, etc.) can also lead to osteoporosis. This bone loss can result in bone fractures, immobility, muscle loss and eventually, frailty. As such it can significantly affect our health, independence, quality of life and life expectancy.[13,14]

While osteoporosis is more common in postmenopausal women, men can also experience bone loss. In order to prevent/reverse osteoporosis, you need to maintain a healthy diet rich in calcium (found in dairy products, sardines, dark leafy greens, enriched flours and cereals, etc.) and vitamin D (fish oil, fish, dairy products, fortified cereals, meat, eggs, mushrooms, etc.). As discussed in the Nutrition chapter, you do not need to take vitamin D or calcium supplements unless your blood results have indicated a need for doing so. Otherwise your body can obtain all the nutrients it requires if you follow a healthy balanced diet. You should engage regularly in weight-bearing exercises (discussed above) in order to put gentle stress on your bones and stimulate bone formation.[15] Make sure to get enough sun exposure as discussed previously. Avoid smoking, since nicotine has a toxic effect on bone cells and also interferes with the body's ability to use estrogen, calcium and vitamin D for the formation of bone cells. Limit your alcohol intake. Alcohol increases calcium loss and can even interfere with bone formation. Furthermore, it can negatively affect your balance and increase your risk of falls and bone fractures.[16]

Note: In addition to following the preceding guidelines, you should discuss osteoporosis with your physician. Your doctor can order a bone density scan for you and determine whether you suffer from osteoporosis. If hormonal deficiencies or medical conditions contribute to bone loss your geriatrician can prescribe necessary medications to prevent or reverse osteoporosis.

Illness

Chronic diseases, infectious diseases and cancer can also lead to pain, fatigue, loss of appetite, impairments, disabilities, and immobility with the end result being frailty. Examples are numerous and we will only discuss a few in this chapter. We have already talked about osteoporosis and its effects on bone and muscle loss. Arthritis also reduces our ability to move and sets the stage for muscle loss. Atherosclerosis, in which clogging of your arteries can deprive muscles (for example in the heart or legs) or brain cells of nutrients and oxygen, can also lead to physical and cognitive impairment. Cognitive impairment can cause a decline in mental processing time and reaction speed and increase the risk of falls.

People suffering from any serious illness are more prone to hospitalizations, bed rest, inactivity, and malnutrition. The consequence is a decline in their ability to perform daily activities, increased reliance on others for assistance, increased risk of social isolation, and of course frailty. Identifying and addressing specific risk factors (such as falls, pain, immobility, malnutrition, delirium, etc.) related to these diseases can reduce the risk of developing frailty. For instance, if you or a loved one suffers from an acute illness, appropriate physical activity in the form of physical therapy and rehabilitation can accelerate recovery and prevent frailty. If you suffer from any chronic disease or cognitive impairment, visit your geriatrician regularly and follow his or her instructions to prevent, slow, or reverse the development of frailty as soon as possible.

Balance Impairment

As a natural part of the aging process as well as due to illnesses (such as osteoarthritis, visual impairment, vestibular dysfunction, cerebrovascular disease, and peripheral neuropathy) and surgical procedures (such as joint replacement) our balance deteriorates. Decreased balance can increase the risk of falls and frailty. Another form of exercise, which is one of my most favorite and the type I highly recommend to my patients, is balance training. Balance training exercises prevent falls and improve concentration. They include activities such as walking backwards, walking sideways, heel walking, toe walking, standing up from a sitting position (rising from a chair) and Tai Chi. Tai Chi is a Chinese martial art discipline described as a mind-body practice. It is a combination of an aerobic workout and resistance training mixed with meditation. Studies have shown that it reduces falls by up to 45% in the elderly and brings about physical and emotional stability. Tai Chi is a low-impact, slow motion exercise, which doesn't put too much strain on joints and bones, and is therefore quite safe. In addition to increasing muscle strength, flexibility, balance, and gait, Tai Chi is very beneficial for several medical conditions such as arthritis (reducing pain and inflammation), osteoporosis (increasing bone density), heart disease (lowering blood pressure, and improving levels of cholesterol, triglycerides, insulin, and C-reactive protein), cancer (improving capacity), hypertension (lowering

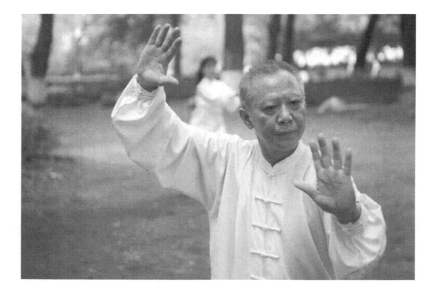

blood pressure), stroke (improving balance), Parkinson's disease (improving balance and walking ability), and depression and anxiety (relieves stress). It is also very useful for preventing lung collapse and decreasing the risk of pneumonia. The AHA/ACSM recommendation is three times per week of balance training exercises. Tai Chi classes are available in many communities. My recommendation is to join a Tai Chi class if you can to socialize, meditate, and exercise your way to better health.

Depression

Researchers have shown that people with psychiatric illnesses such as depression are at a higher risk of developing frailty.[17] As we saw in the Mental Health chapter, emotional stress can have negative effects on our physical and mental health. It can interfere with our sleep, speed of recovery from illness, appetite, concentration, focus, and cognitive functions. People who suffer from depression and anxiety are also more prone to developing medical illnesses. In previous chapters we discussed many methods of alleviating stress, depression and anxiety caused by life events.

It is worth mentioning that depression and other mental disorders could also have an underlying biological cause. Chemical imbalances in the brain involving neurotransmitters, hormonal changes due to thyroid problems, menopause, or other factors as well as genetic factors can cause depression. Depression can also be caused by medications, especially blood pressure medications and sleeping pills. If you believe you are depressed, you should discuss this issue with your geriatrician and a geriatric psychologist or psychiatrist. If they determine that your depression is due to chemical imbalances, they can prescribe anti-depressant medications for you. While anti-depressants alleviate depression caused by chemical imbalances, they only help some with depression caused by medications, hormonal imbalances, genetic factors, or life events.

As a word of caution, I have noticed many physicians over prescribing anti-depressants or anti-anxiety medications to the elderly without identifying the root cause of their mental illness. In many cases these medications can cause more harm by resulting in further loss of appetite, immobility, confusion and delirium. It is therefore vital to research the cause of depression and other mental disorders before prescribing such medications to the elderly. Be sure to talk to your physician in detail about why they are prescribing a particular drug and what the alternatives are so that you can make an informed decision about it.

Take Home Message

Timely intervention and aggressive treatment to maintain and hopefully restore physical activity and cognitive reserves are essential in order to prevent, slow, or reverse the development of frailty. You can live a longer healthy, happy, and independent existence if you incorporate the following into your life:

- A healthy diet
- A regimen of fun exercises
- A set of good lifestyle choices
- Education about the causes, prevention and early detection of frailty
- Proper treatment
- Routine visits to your geriatrician or other health care provider
- Engagement in fun social activities to prevent isolation and depression

EXERCISES

I. Older adults need to perform mild aerobic (endurance) exercises five days a week for a minimum of 30 minutes without stopping. Examples include:

- Walking
- Swimming
- Dancing
- Gardening (such as pushing a lawn mower)
- Vacuuming or other house cleaning chores
- Biking
- Yoga

II. Older adults need to perform strength training (strenuous) exercises at least twice per week. They should do 8-10 of such exercises. Each exercise should be repeated 8-12 times during each session. Examples include:
   • Light lifting of weights
   • Working with resistance bands
   • Using body weight for resistance in exercises such as push-ups, pull ups and sit ups
   • Climbing stairs
   • Chair squats

III. Older adults need to perform balance training exercises three times per week. Examples include:
   • Walking backwards
   • Sideways walking
   • Heel walking
   • Toe walking
   • Standing up from a sitting position (rising from a chair)
   • Tai Chi

Here are Some Exercises I Highly Recommend to My Patients:

1. **Arm Chair Push**

   This is a very useful exercise to strengthen your arms. This exercise is especially beneficial for people who use a walker. One of the big issues we see as geriatricians is that many patients are unable to use their walker because their arms are weak. Try to do this exercise twice per day and repeat 10 times each time.

The following exercise pictures were taken by Dr. Ayati in collaboration with Jonathan Ray Mendoza (Physical Therapist)

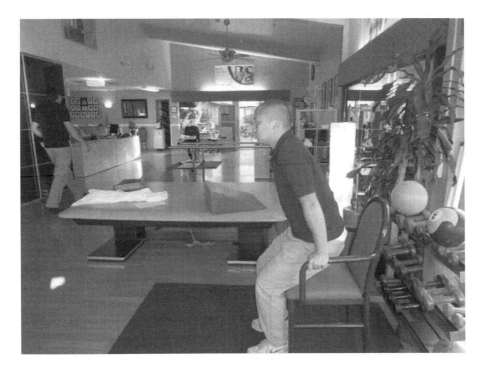

2. **Long ARC Quad**

This is a very useful exercise for strengthening your knees, especially the tendons. This is also useful for people who are suffering from knee osteoarthritis pain. You need to sit on a chair and straighten each leg, holding it for 6 seconds. Repeat 20 times for each leg and do two sessions per day.

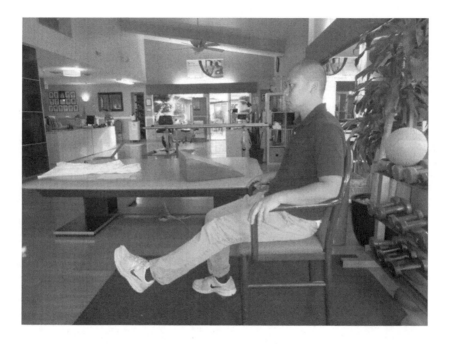

3. **Sitting Chair Flexion**

This is another useful exercise I recommend to everyone in any age group (preferably on a daily basis). This exercise will improve your lower extremities' strength and flexibility and improve your balance. You can do this exercise anytime even when you are watching TV or talking to your friends. You need to sit relaxed on a chair and raise your knee up while your knee is bent. Repeat 20 times for each side and repeat at least twice per day.

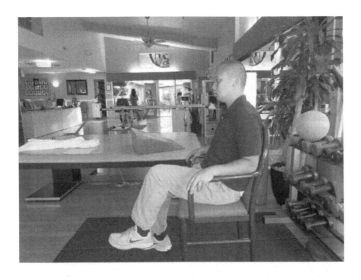

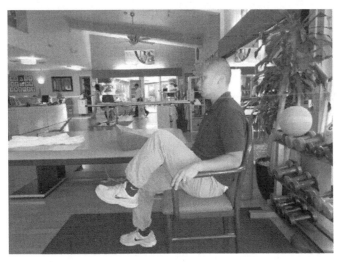

4. **Legs Apart**

This exercise helps strengthen your pelvic area. Sit straight and move your legs widely apart and then bring them back together. Repeat 20 times and perform two sessions per day.

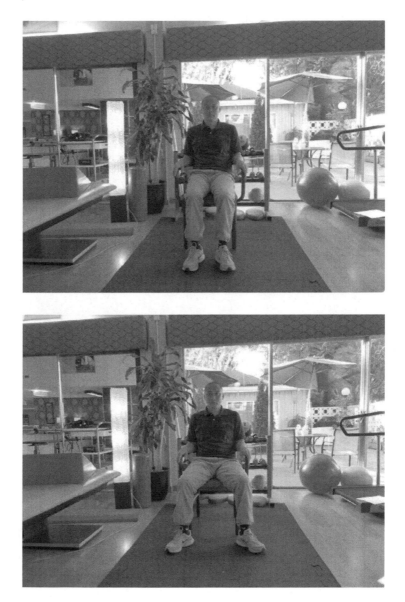

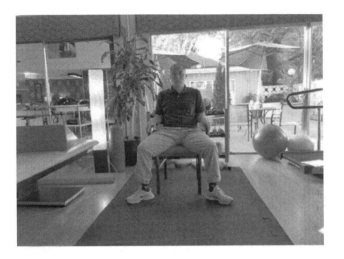

5. **Hip "I Love a Parade" Lift**

This is a great exercise in order to increase your hip strength and for prevention of falls. You can do this while holding the back of a chair or without it. Lift each knee as high as possible four times and repeat the same exercise on your other knee.

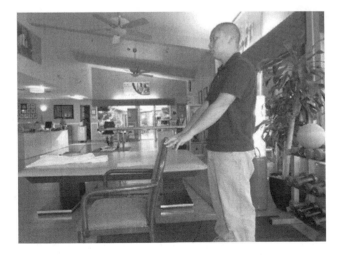

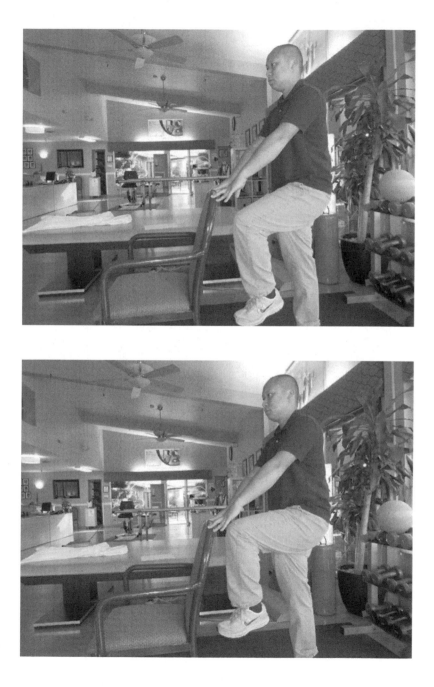

6. **Knee Bend**

This exercise strengthens your knees and improves balance. Hold the back of a chair and keeping both feet on the floor slowly bend your knees. Repeat 10 times and perform two sessions per day.

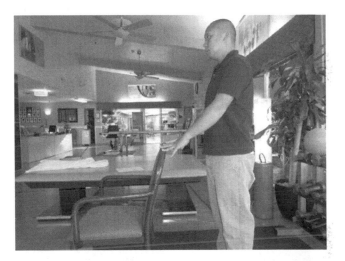

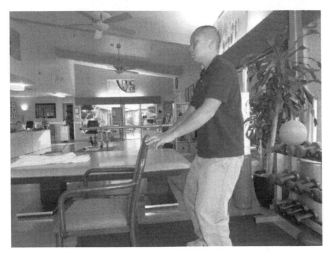

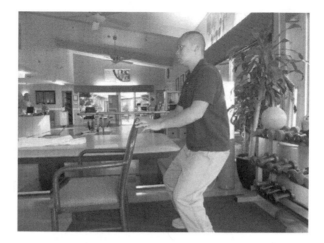

7. **Hip Backward Kick**

Hold the back of a chair. Part your legs slightly while keeping your toes pointed forward. Slowly extend one leg backward while keeping your knees straight. Make sure you are not leaning forward. Switch to the other leg and repeat. Perform this exercise 10 times on each leg and repeat twice per day.

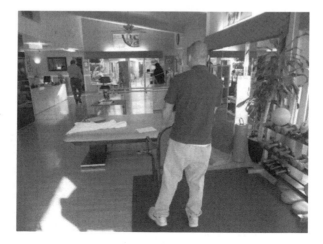

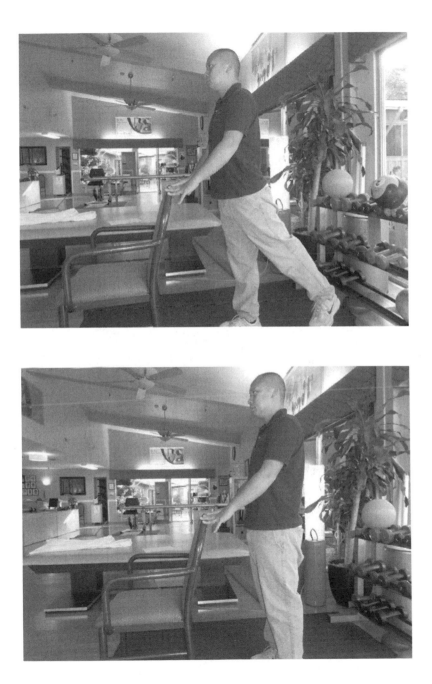

8. **Hip Side Kick**

Hold the back of a chair. Part your legs slightly while keeping your toes pointed forward. Swing a leg out to the side while keeping your knee straight. Make sure you are not leaning forward. Switch to the other leg and repeat. Perform this exercise 10 times on each leg and repeat twice per day.

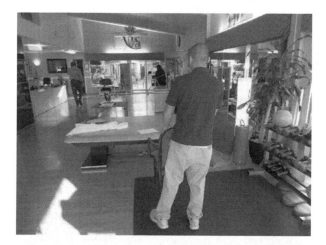

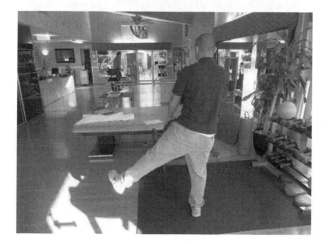

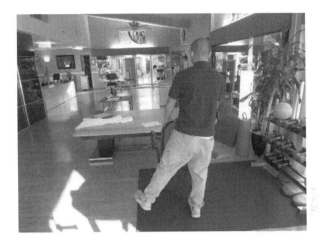

9. **Hamstring Strengthening**

Hold the back of a chair. Lift your right heel toward your buttocks. Repeat the same exercise with the left heel. Repeat this exercise 10 times twice per day.

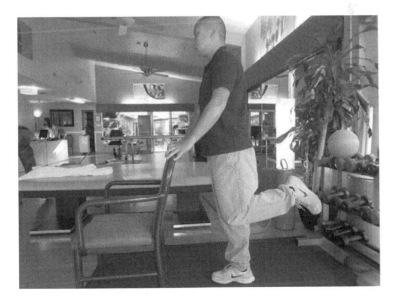

ACTION PLAN

1. If you suffer from lack of energy, overtiredness, feebleness, lack of strength, inability, dizziness, loss of balance, recent history of falls and/ or lack of appetite discuss this with your physician as soon as possible

2. Show the list of enclosed exercises in this chapter to your physician and with his or her guidance perform a few for a period of one month. Do you feel any difference in your health?

3. Ask your doctor whether you need to have a bone density scan

REFERENCES

1. Frailty in elderly people. Clegg A, Young J, Iliffe S, Rikkert MO, Rockwood K, Lancet. 2013;381(9868):752-62.

2. Untangling the concepts of disability, frailty, and comorbidity: implications for improved targeting and care. Fried, LP; Ferrucci L, Darer J, Williamson JD, Anderson G, J Gerontol A Biol Sci Med Sci. 2004; 59 (3): 255–63.

3. Life-space constriction, development of frailty, and the competing risk of mortality: the Women's Health And Aging Study I. Xue, QL; Fried LP, Glass TA, Laffan A, Chaves PH, Am J Epidemiol. 2008;167 (2): 240–8.

4. Impact of anemia and cardiovascular disease on frailty status of community-dwelling older women: the Women's Health and Aging Studies I and II. Chaves, PH; Semba RD, Leng SX, Woodman RC, Ferrucci L, Guralnik JM, Fried LP, J Gerontol A Biol Sci Med Sci. 2005;60 (6): 729–35.

5. Phenotype of frailty: characterization in the women's health and aging studies. Bandeen-Roche, K; Xue QL., Ferrucci L, Walston J, Guralnik JM, Chaves P, Zeger SL, Fried LP, J Gerontol A Biol Sci Med Sci. 2006;61 (3): 262–6.

6. Malnutrition in older adults - urgent need for action: a plea for improving the nutritional situation of older adults. Volkert D, Gerontology. 2013;59(4):328-33.

7. Loss of appetite in elderly people in the community and its relationship with functional capacity. Serra Prat M, Fernández X, Ribó L, Palomera E, Papiol M, Serra P, Med Clin (Barc). 2008;130(14):531-3.

8. Sarcopenia. Morley JE, Baumgartner RN, Roubenoff R, Mayer J, Nair KS, J Lab Clin Med. 2001;137(4):231-43.

9. Optimum Sports Nutrition. Colgan M, New York: Advanced Research Press. 1993.

10. Resistance training, sarcopenia, and the mitochondrial theory of aging. Johnston AP, De Lisio M, Parise G, Appl Physiol Nutr Metab. 2008;33(1):191–199.

11. Dose-response issues concerning physical activity and health: an evidence-based symposium. Kesaniemi YK, Danforth E Jr, Jensen MD, Kopelman PG, Lefèbvre P, Reeder BA. Med Sci Sports Exerc. 2001;33(6 Suppl):S351-8.

12. Physical activity and public health: updated recommendation for adults from the American College of Sports Medicine and the American Heart Association. Haskell WL, Lee IM, Pate RR, Powell KE, Blair SN, Franklin BA, Macera CA, Heath GW, Thompson PD, Bauman A. Med Sci Sports Exerc. 2007;39(8):1423-34.

13. Frailty and fracture, disability, and falls: a multiple country study from the global longitudinal study of osteoporosis in women. Tom SE, Adachi JD, Anderson FA Jr, Boonen S, Chapurlat RD, Compston JE, Cooper C, Gehlbach SH, Greenspan SL, Hooven FH, Nieves JW, Pfeilschifter J, Roux C, Silverman S, Wyman A, LaCroix AZ; GLOW Investigators. J Am Geriatr Soc. 2013;61(3):327-34.

14. The effect of treatments for osteoporosis on mortality. Grey A, Bolland MJ, Osteoporos Int. 2013;24(1):1-6.

15. Resistance Training Is an Effective Tool against Metabolic and Frailty Syndromes. Sundell J, Adv Prev Med. 2011;2011:984683.

16. Role of obesity, alcohol and smoking on bone health. Fini M, Salamanna F, Veronesi F, Torricelli P, Nicolini A, Benedicenti S, Carpi A, Giavaresi G, Front Biosci (Elite Ed). 2012;4:2686-706.

17. Psychiatric illness in relation to frailty in community-dwelling elderly people without dementia: a report from the Canadian Study of Health and Aging. Andrew MK, Rockwood K, Can J Aging. 2007;26(1):33-8.

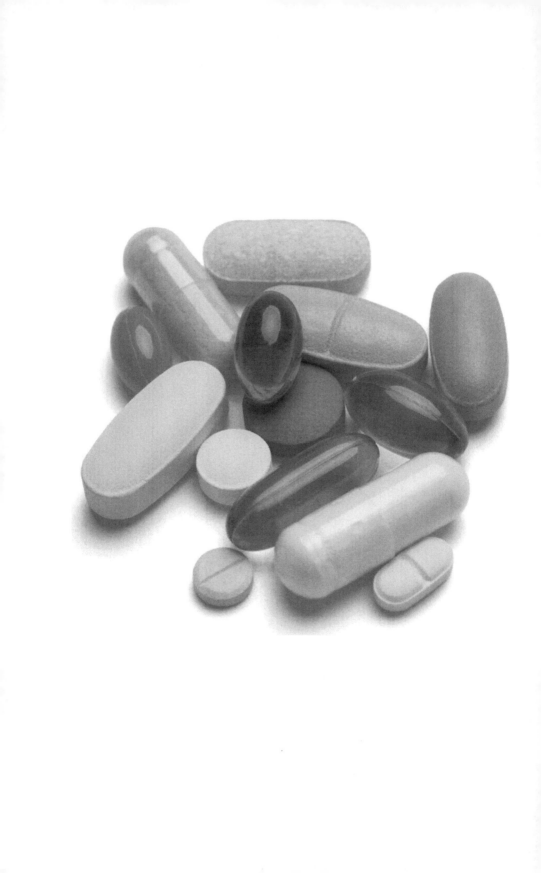

Chapter 4

Overmedication (Polypharmacy)

Questions to Ask Yourself

1. Do you have a complete list of all the medications (prescriptions, over the counter, supplements and herbal remedies) you take, including the reason for taking them, any side effects they might cause, and the side effects they have caused you?

2. Do you have a list of all the medications you have been instructed to discontinue? Have you included the reason(s) you were told to discontinue these medications and the side effects they caused you?

3. Do you ask your physicians to explain why they have prescribed new medications for you and the possible side effects they might cause?

4. Have you asked your doctor to ensure that the new medication he or she is prescribing for you does not interact with your existing medications?

5. Each time a new medication has been prescribed for you by another provider, have you discussed the possible consequences with your geriatrician?

6. Do you get your prescription filled at the same pharmacy each time you have a new medication?

7. Do you present a complete list of all of your medications, OTC drugs, supplements & herbal remedies to your specialists and primary care provider?

8. Do your discard the medications you are no longer taking?

9. Do you drink alcohol while taking prescription medications, OTC drugs, supplements and herbal remedies?

A couple of years ago, I visited a patient at a skilled nursing facility who had fallen at home and ended up with a broken hip. After thorough examination it turned out that for months the patient had been suffering from a chronic medical condition called Restless Leg Syndrome (RLS). RLS is a neurological disorder characterized by unpleasant sensations (such as throbbing, creeping, or pulling) in the legs and an uncontrollable urge to continuously move them. Symptoms primarily occur at night while a person is lying down and trying to relax and sleep. As a result most people with RLS suffer from sleep deprivation, which can lead to exhaustion, fatigue, lack of concentration, impaired memory and depression. While suffering from RLS the patient had visited his primary care physician on multiple occasions to seek treatment. Unfortunately, instead of treating the RLS, the provider decided to treat the patient's depression (which was caused by prolonged RLS and lack of sleep) and prescribed him antidepressants (called Selective Serotonin Reuptake Inhibitors or SSRIs). While taking the antidepressants his leg cramps got worse and as a result of severe exhaustion, fatigue, and lack of sleep he became disoriented and fell. Once he ended up at the skilled nursing facility, where he remained immobilized for a large part of three months, his quality of life suffered more. He was in pain, lost his appetite and a significant amount of weight, and became severely depressed. His family members reported that they could not believe he was the same person they had known for years. Fortunately, after he discontinued the antidepressants wrongly prescribed to him and his broken hip healed, we were able to slowly reverse his condition, and he fully recovered. This tragedy could have been avoided if his RLS was treated in the first place and he was not prescribed antidepressants. Most over the counter medication (OTC) and SSRI antidepressants worsen RLS.

Another patient I recently visited at a skilled nursing facility suffered from a fall and as a result brain hemorrhage. Five months prior to his fall he was diagnosed with mild short-term memory loss (called Mild Cognitive Insufficiency or MCI). MCI is not dementia, although MCI may increase the risk of later progressing to dementia, caused by Alzheimer's disease or other neurological conditions. However, people with MCI may never get worse, and may eventually get better. The patient's physician decided to treat the patient's mild cognitive insufficiency by prescribing cholinesterase inhibitor (a type of drug approved for Alzheimer's disease) for him. However, cholinesterase inhibitors aren't recommended for routine treatment of MCI because they don't appear to provide lasting benefit (http://tinyurl.com/nmrolvm). Once the patient started taking this medication at night he began having vivid dreams. He reported the side effect to his physician. Instead of stopping this medication, the physician put the patient on sleeping aid medication. As a result of taking both the cholinesterase inhibitor and the sleeping pills, the patient's vivid dreams now became delusional-like thoughts, and he developed anxiety at night-time, waking up multiple times with nightmare attacks. Once again he reported the problem to his physician and his doctor then decided to prescribe a stronger sleep medication for him. As a result the patient ended up falling and hitting his head, which caused a brain hemorrhage. Unfortunately, the patient passed away. Had his physician stopped cholinesterase inhibitor in the first place instead of prescribing sleeping medication for him, the patient would have been able to prevent the fall and the resulting brain hemorrhage and all the tragic complications which had followed.

Every patient who walks into my clinic is on some sort of medication. Seniors are the largest consumers of prescription and over the counter medications. Over 40 percent of the elderly take at least five medications.[1-2] This is considered a form of overmedication: the technical term is *polypharmacy*. Polypharmacy is a problem because it can result in dangerous drug interactions and cause serious and even fatal side effects.[3-5] These adverse effects include heart failure, seizures, disorientation, confusion, weakness, sedation, falls, fractures, hypotension, incontinence, electrolytic disorders, anxiety, delirium, mental decline, blurred vision, constipation, GI bleeding, and loss of appetite.[6] Adverse drug events (ADEs) account for a large number of hospitalizations (5-26% of all geriatric admissions) and deaths among the elderly. And ADEs have a high cost associated with them. In nursing homes for every 1 dollar spent on medications, a staggering 1.33 dollars in healthcare resources is consumed in the treatment of drug-related morbidity and mortality.

Here's a common way polypharmacy occurs. Seniors often have multiple health issues and see different specialists. Each physician relies on their patient's information to prescribe the necessary medication(s) for them. However, too often, the patients forget to disclose the name of all the medications (including the OTC medications, supplements and herbal remedies) they take and all the illnesses they suffer from. The specialists might therefore prescribe medications to them which could lead to harmful drug interactions or inactivate the effect of the other medications they are on.

Therefore, it is crucial that you do the following:

- Keep a list of the names of all of your illnesses and the medications (including the dosage) you are taking for each and **share the list with all your physicians and your pharmacist**.

- Update your list each time a new medication or dosage is prescribed or if you have been asked to discontinue a medication. Write down the side-effects you experienced with each and the reason why it was replaced by another medication or discontinued.

- Question your physicians thoroughly about each of the new medications they prescribe and ask them to ensure that they do not interact with or inactivate your existing medications.

- Also make sure you understand clearly the doctor's instructions about each new medication she or he is prescribing for you. Write down the reason you need to take the medication and directions for use (the dosage, when you need to take each dose, and how) as well as all the possible side effects it might cause. Repeat this to the doctor before you leave the office.
- Fill out your prescription at the same pharmacy each time you have a new medication. That way your pharmacist will have your complete medication profile and will be able to detect drug interactions.

Specialists are physicians with expertise in a specific field. That is why you visit a cardiologist when you have heart problems or a neurologist if you suffer from neurological issues. Note that specialists are not trained on all medications and their side effects or their interactions with other drugs. Therefore, even if you disclose a list of all of your medications to your specialists they might not know if they could pose problems. Let me give you a hypothetical example here.

Helen is a 60 year old accountant who visits her endocrinologist for hormonal deficiencies—he prescribes a hormone to her. Then, she sees a GI specialist who tells her that she is developing an ulcer and should take proton pump inhibiters to lower her stomach acid. Next, Helen goes to a psychiatrist, who prescribes an antidepressant to her. She then sees a cardiologist, who prescribes blood pressure lowering medication to her and advises her to take an aspirin every day. In addition to these specialists, Helen visits her primary physician, who notes she is slightly above the normal range for her cholesterol and puts her on cholesterol-lowering medication. On top of that she has been advised by one of her friends to drink lots of chamomile tea and she read on the Internet that she should take over-the-counter garlic pills as a "natural" way to lower her cholesterol and blood pressure. To make things worse Helen takes all of these medications with grapefruit juice since she thinks taking an extra amount of vitamin C is beneficial to her health and she loves grapefruit juice.

Well, the grapefruit juice neutralizes the effect of a few of her medications (including the cholesterol-lowering medication). And then the grapefruit juice, garlic, chamomile and the blood lowering medication combine to cause a sharp drop in her blood pressure with dire consequences. Furthermore, the garlic causes additional GI upset. The anti-hypertension medication that was prescribed to her causes depression, and she already is depressed. The aspirin will worsen her stomach ulcer and can lead to bleeding. As you can see, the different specialists prescribed medications in their field of specialty to her and failed to foresee the possible side effects these medications might present. Many medications she ends up taking either make her other symptoms worse or have a counter effect on the ones she is already taking. And this goes on and on until Helen gets seriously ill.

Another major concern is when physicians prescribe medications for patients to treat the side effects of one or more current drugs they are taking. In this case, an undesirable side effect is misinterpreted as a medical condition and results in a new prescription, which could result in additional side effects. This is called a **drug cascade syndrome** and is a major reason why 4.5 million Americans (mostly people aged 65 and older) visit the emergency rooms and physician offices each year (http://tinyurl.com/kzwys9u). To put this simply, a patient goes to a specialist office with an illness and is given a medication (let's call it medication A). Medication A has a side effect that causes another illness and now the patient unaware that the medication A is the problem visits another specialist and is given medication B. Medication B now results in a new side effect, which sends the patient to yet another specialist for the new illness the patient is experiencing and is given medication C. And this cascade continues until the patient ends up with many unnecessary and harmful medications causing adverse side effects.

To avoid experiencing a drug cascade like this, be sure to do the following:

- Before you take any medication, make sure your physician cites the possible side effects to you.
- If you experience any of those side effects, **visit the same doctor as soon as possible** so that your medication can

be altered. It is imperative that you see the same physician if you can. Changing your physician increases the chances of a drug cascade episode because the new physician may be less aware of your medication and illness history. Also, do not discontinue the medication until you see your physician. It could be even more harmful if you stop your medications without consulting your physician first.

• Make sure you discard the medications you are no longer taking. Storing many different types of medication bottles can result in confusion and increase your chances of taking the wrong one. For a guide on how to safely discard your unwanted medication refer to: http://tinyurl.com/okx25k3.

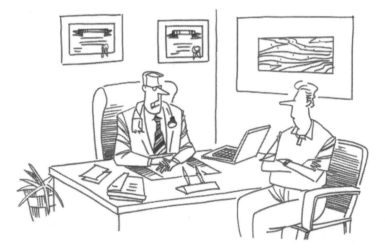

"The problem is that you're overmedicated.
Luckily there are drugs that can help with that."

Of course drug cascade syndrome can happen even if you visit the same doctor. Here is an example. Carl, a 52 year old engineer, visits his doctor at the beginning of the year and complains about insomnia and asks for a sleeping medication. His doctor prescribes it for Carl. A month later Carl goes back to his doctor and complains about fatigue (which is a side effect of the sleeping medication Carl is on) and asks for a medication to make him feel less tired. The doctor advises against it and instead recommends that Carl discontinue his sleeping pill or lower its dose. Carl, however, insists on staying on it (since it has been helping him to sleep) and in addition insists on taking another medication to feel less tired during the day. The doctor then reluctantly prescribes a stimulant for Carl to take during the day. A month later Carl goes back to his doctor's office and complains about heart palpitation (a side effect of the stimulant he is taking). The doctor again advises Carl to discontinue both the sleeping medication and his stimulant. Instead, Carl keeps on insisting that he needs both medications and yet another drug to control the heart palpitation. This time the doctor prescribes a beta blocker for Carl to control his heart rate. During his next visit Carl complains of depression (a side effect of the beta blocker) and asks for an antidepressant. After Carl takes the antidepressant he goes back to his doctor and complains about weight gain (a side effect of the antidepressant). This continues until Carl ends up with multiple medications and many side effects. The moral of this story is that taking a medication is not always a wise decision and can end up causing more harm than benefit.

Make sure to discuss all of your medications with your geriatrician. We saw in previous chapters that as we age our body's physiology changes. For example, absorption of drugs through our digestive system can be altered. Our liver function decreases, and it becomes harder for our body to metabolize and eliminate drugs. Changes in our circulatory and nervous systems affect our reactions to drugs.[7-8] Therefore, we might need lower or higher doses of medications compared to other age groups. And there are medications that while working perfectly well for younger adults, should not be prescribed for the geriatric population. Examples include antihistamines, which are available over the counter (can cause confusion, constipation, urination problems, dry mouth and blurred vision), muscle relaxants (can cause grogginess, confusion, constipation, dry mouth, problems with urination and increased risk of falls), opioid pain relievers (can cause confusion, hallucinations, falls, and seizures), and long-lasting Non-Steroidal Anti-Inflammatory Drugs (NSAIDs) (can increase the risk of indigestion, ulcers, bleeding in the stomach or colon, affect the kidneys, and increase blood pressure). Geriatricians are specialists in elderly healthcare. They have the necessary training on age-associated changes affecting the metabolism and absorption of drugs and are thus best suited to adjust your medications. **Therefore, make sure to visit or at least inform your geriatrician**

each time a new drug is prescribed to you. Note however that geriatricians (like other specialists) are not God. If you suspect that your geriatrician is prescribing too many medications to you and that you are suffering from many side effects, make an appointment with another geriatrician for a second opinion.

Similarly to certain prescription drugs, OTC medications, supplements and herbal remedies can cause sleepiness, dizziness, slower physical reactions, disorientation, problems remembering things or paying attention, and delirium. Sometimes, these symptoms could be mistaken to be indicative of Alzheimer's disease, even though they are caused by the medications. Therefore, my advice is to refrain from taking *any* OTC medications, supplements and herbal remedies, no matter how much you have heard about them in the media, unless directed by your doctor. The global vitamin and supplement market is currently worth $68 billion USD (Euromonitor). Over 100,000 OTC medications exist in the market.[9] There is a vast marketing campaign at every corner enticing people to consume them regardless of the fact that there is no evidence indicating their benefits. As we discussed in previous chapters, supplements can't replace proper nutrition and should not be taken unless a blood test analysis ordered by your physicians justifies prescribing them. Remember too that supplements and herbal remedies can interfere with prescription drugs and cause severe health problems including organ damage or even death. For a list of some commonly used supplements and their adverse effects refer to

Table 1. While prescription drugs are stringently regulated by the U.S. Food and Drug Administration (FDA), OTCs, supplements and herbal remedies are not. As such the manufacturers of such supplements do not have to prove their safety or efficacy in any format (http://tinyurl.com/cj6fvlv). Hence, be very cautious before you add them to your diet.

Table 1

Herbal Medication	Potential Benefit	Side Effects	Possible Interaction with Other Medications
COQ10	• Antioxidant • Help for heart failure symptoms in some patients • Possible anti-cancer	• Insomnia • Elevated liver enzymes	• Blood pressure medications • Chemotherapy medications • Warfarin (blood thinner)
Garlic	• Lowering blood pressure • Lowering cholesterol • Blood thinner	• Stomach upset • Diarrhea • Lightheadedness • Eczema • Rash • Lower blood glucose (sugar)	• Blood thinner medications • Diabetic medications • HIV medications
Echinacea	• Immune system stimulant • Treatment of common cold • Burns or wounds	• Headache • Dizziness • Nausea • Constipation	• Steroid medications • Immune suppressant medications

Ginseng	• Reducing body stress • Cancer prevention • Improving physical and mental performance	• Allergic reaction • High blood pressure • Diarrhea • Lower blood sugar	• Diabetic medications • Blood thinner • Heart medications
Glucosamine	• Treatment of osteoarthritis	• Nausea • Diarrhea • Heartburn	• Insulin • Blood thinner
St. John's Wort	Alleviates: • Depression • Anxiety • Insomnia • Fibromyalgia • Nerve pain • Irritable bowel syndrome	• Irritation • Stomach upset • Dizziness • Dry mouth • Skin allergic reaction and rash • Sleep disturbance	• Blood thinners • Heart medication especially anti-arrhythmia medication • Antidepressant medication

Finally, remember that drinking alcohol with prescription medications, OTC drugs, supplements and herbal remedies is another source of serious problems for the elderly (and for others as well). For instance, it is unsafe to drink alcohol if you are taking medications for sleep, pain, anxiety or depression. Also, keep in mind that even if you take a medication in the morning it is most likely not safe to drink alcohol in the afternoon or with dinner. As we learned, it is harder for our body to metabolize and eliminate drugs as we age. Consequently, medications remain in our system much longer.

Take Home Message

With aging, the risk of having one or more chronic diseases requiring multiple medications increases. However, taking several drugs simultaneously raises your chance of suffering from adverse drug events and unsafe drug interactions. In order to protect yourself:

1. Keep an up-to-date and thorough list of all your medications
2. Share them with *all* your physicians and pharmacists
3. Fill all your prescriptions at the same pharmacy
4. Consult your geriatrician each time a new medication is prescribed for you
5. Refrain from taking OTC, supplements and herbal remedies

And remember that taking a medication is not always a wise choice: any therapeutic benefit can be outweighed by the potential for drug cascade syndrome and other harmful interaction effects. Take only what you truly need.

MEHRDAD AYATI AND AREZOU AZARANI

This is a letter from one of my very special patients and friends,
Dr. Martin Katz

Martin Katz: Director of Pharmaceutical Research and Sculptor

As a Director of Pharmaceutical Research for over thirty years,
I am fully aware of our incredible achievements in medication
and the benefits they have provided for our health and longevity.

Certainly the efficiency of our organs will diminish with age and our
genetic inheritance will play a major role in setting the rate and time.
We are fortunate that we can now ameliorate, delay and even substitute
for many of these changes.

So you now have an opportunity and an obligation to take advantage
of these wonderful medical advances to enjoy a healthier, joyful,
positive and more fulfilling life.

But, do we really need all the medications we have personally
accumulated over the years?
Are they an accumulation of needless and possibly harmful medications
that were possibly prescribed for some minor or acute episode that you
have maintained, perpetuated and turned into a chronic ailment.

Have you actively tried to change your sedentary lifestyle and get rid of
some of those drugs? There are so many opportunities

Mental Activity - The brain, even after sixty, if it is fed a diet of complexity,
newness and problem solving can flower and bloom.
Physical Activity - Get off that couch, turn off the TV! At least go for a
walk.
Social Interaction - You must have friends, a partner. Join a senior center,
a club, your worship center. Get out of the house.
Diet Control - Endless opportunities

At 87, I belong to two senior centers that provide wonderful social
interaction,

*friends, trips and activities. I go to the gym twice a week.
My avocation as a sculptor has provided me with a "new" life with
physical activity, mental challenge, social interaction and friends.
And the number of pills that I have reduced or dropped is amazing!*

*My Mantra
You all have an interest or hobby or activity that you wanted to do instead
of working.
But if you don't join a class or a group, you are not going to do it.
No matter how self-motivated I am, if I don't put it on the calendar,
I will find a million excuses to put off an activity or a hobby.*

GO DO IT!

This is a sculpture by Dr. Katz at the age of 87

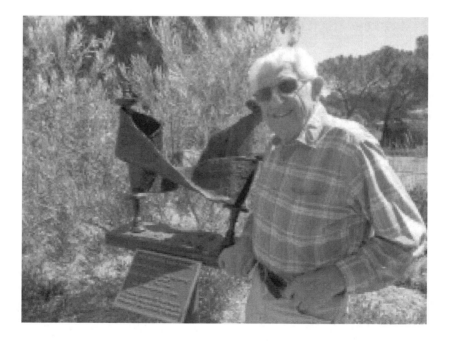

ACTION PLAN

1. Dispose of your unwanted drugs

2. Make sure to update the list of all your medications (including over the counter medications, supplements and herbal remedies) and include the reason(s) for taking them and their side effects. Bring it with you to your physician(s) during each visit.

3. Make a list of all the medications you have been instructed to discontinue. Include the reason(s) you were told to discontinue each and the side effects they caused you. Bring this list to your physician(s) during each visit.

4. Each time a new medication has been prescribed for you make sure to inform or visit your geriatrician.

REFERENCES

1. Medication use among older Australian veterans and war widows. Byles JE, Heinze R, Nair BK, Parkinson L, Intern Med J. 2003;33:388–92.

2. Use of medications and polypharmacy are increasing among the elderly. Linjakumpu T, Hartikainen S, Klaukka T, Veijola J, Kivelä SL, Isoaho R, J Clin Epidemiol. 2002;55(8):809-17.

3. Analysis of the direct cost of adverse drug reactions in hospitalised patients. Bordet R, Gautier S, Le Louet H, Dupuis B, Caron J, Eur J Clin Pharmacol. 2001;56(12):935-41.

4. Adverse drug reactions as cause of visit to the emergency department: incidence, features and outcomes. Zanocchi M, Tibaldi V, Amati D, Francisetti F, Martinelli E, Gonella M, Cerrato F, Ponte E, Luppino A, Bardelli B, Canadè A, Gariglio F, Moiraghi C, Molaschi M, Recenti Prog Med. 2006;97(7-8):381-8.

5. Incidence and preventability of adverse drug events among older persons in the ambulatory setting. Gurwitz JH, Field TS, Harrold LR, Rothschild J, Debellis K, Seger AC, Cadoret C, Fish LS, Garber L, Kelleher M, Bates DW, JAMA. 2003;289:1107-1116.

6. Médicaments et personnes âgées. Barbeau G, Guimond J, Mallet L, Edisem-Maloine, St-Hyacinthe, 1991.

7. Clinical implications of changes in hepatic drug metabolism in older people. Hilmer SN, Shenfield GM, Le Couteur DG, Ther Clin Risk Manag. 2005; 1(2): 151–156.

8. Age-related changes in pharmacokinetics and pharmacodynamics: basic principles and practical applications. A A Mangoni and S H D Jackson, Br J Clin Pharmacol. 2004 January; 57(1): 6–14.

9. Over-the-counter medication use in older adults. Rolita L, Freedman M, J Gerontol Nurs. 2008; 34: 8–17.

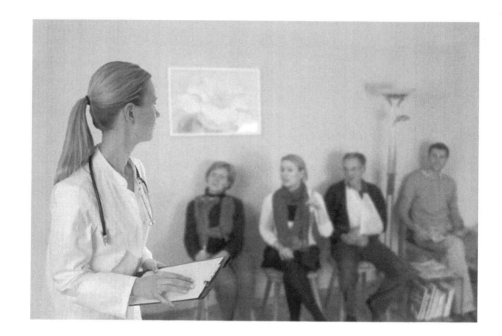

Chapter 5

How to Find a Geriatrician

Questions to Ask Yourself

1. Do you currently have a geriatrician?

2. If not, do you know where or how to find a good geriatrician?

3. Describe your ideal geriatrician (for example, someone who listens to you, someone who is available to you 24/7, someone who cares about you, someone who takes the time to explain things to you thoroughly, etc.):

Answer the following questions if you already have a geriatrician:

4. When you visit your geriatrician do you go to their office prepared with an updated list of your medications, medical conditions, the names of your primary care physician and all the specialists you see, and a copy of all your test results?

5. Do you prepare a list of questions and concerns which you need to discuss with your geriatrician before your visit?

6. Do you make notes during your visit with your geriatrician, including all his or her advice and instructions (and do you read those notes when you return home)?

7. Do you feel nervous or intimidated when you see your geriatrician? Why?

8. Do you trust your geriatrician? Does he or she listen to you carefully, give you advice and instructions and make sure you understood everything that was discussed during your visit?

A few months back I was with a patient in my exam room when I overhead loud shouting noises coming from the reception area. When my patient and I could no longer ignore the profanity exchanges I apologized to my patient and went to check what was going on. I recognized one of my patients, who was at this point highly agitated and out of control, screaming at the top of his lungs at my receptionist. I asked what was going on and the receptionist told me that this patient walked into the clinic and demanded to be seen by me right away without any prior appointment. I tried to calm down the patient and see what was upsetting him this much. He said that he had called my clinic for his routine checkup and was told that the waiting list was six months long. He told me this was insane and highly bureaucratic. "Who the hell did I think I was!" he asked. I explained to him that the sheer number of patients with highly complicated medical conditions does not allow us to see more than 8-10 patients per day. To be fully effective, geriatricians need to spend approximately 45 minutes with each patient to thoroughly evaluate their health, complications, medications, answer their questions, address their family members' concerns, etc. I further explained that on a routine basis I have patients complaining to me that when they see their primary care physician or specialists they hardly spend 15 minutes with them. This short visit does not allow them to fully address their medical conditions and concerns. The patient agreed with me that this is indeed why he is drawn to my clinic. I give him a chance to talk, I listen to him, and give him my full attention so that once he leaves my clinic he feels satisfied and content with the quality of the visit. Convinced by my explanation, the patient apologized and agreed to make an appointment to see me in six months unless an emergency visit was needed.

My patients tell me that it is very hard to find a geriatrician, let alone find one they like. They don't have a lot of choices. And when they find one they like, the waiting time to see the doctor is very long. I agree with them. In 2011 the first of 78 million baby boomers started turning 65. And for the next 18 years, they will be turning 65 at a rate of approximately 8,000 per day! About 60 percent of the baby boomers have been diagnosed with at least one chronic disease, with the most common being arthritis, diabetes, heart disease and hypertension. And as we saw in the last chapter, many are taking multiple prescription medications. As a result, geriatricians need to spend a lot of time with each patient to thoroughly understand and assist them with their medical needs. Therefore, to no surprise, geriatricians can't fit too many patients into their day and practice. All these factors are leading to a shortage of geriatricians. However, they are still out there, and you can find one you like, respect, and form a long term relationship with. In this chapter we will discuss a few tips on how to find a good geriatrician, as well as how to interact with them and what to expect from them.

First, keep in mind that geriatricians are specialists. They provide comprehensive care for older adults suffering from complications related to physical and mental health. Additionally, they are specialized in preventative care, rehabilitation, management of patients in long-term care settings, end of life issues, and complex psycho-social, ethical, legal, and economic issues pertinent to the elderly. Consequently, you do not need to see them often. In fact, you should mainly see a geriatrician in the following circumstances:

- if you have been diagnosed with a new chronic condition, cancer or mental disorder;
- every time you have been prescribed a new medication by other physicians (as discussed in the previous chapter);
- once a year to make sure that your chronic conditions are under check;
- once a month if you are in a long-term care institution.

How do you go about finding a "good" geriatrician? Well, you can ask your friends, colleagues, family members, senior care centers, or specialists if they know a good geriatrician in your community that they trust and respect. As I mentioned above, do not get discouraged if these providers have a long waiting list. Actually, your primary care physician should have a list of geriatricians practicing in your community. You can ask him or her to refer you to one for a consult. Once you have found one and made an appointment, be sure to prepare the following documents before your visit. The more prepared you are, the more productive your visit will be.

- Prepare a list of all your medical problems and history. Include the names of your primary care physician and all the specialists you see. If you have laboratory tests or radiology results, always bring a copy. The doctor might ask you to sign a release form to get your medical records from your primary care provider. However, that takes much longer.

- As discussed in the previous chapter, you should always have an updated list of all of your medications. Make sure you list the ones you are taking currently as well as the ones you took previously but your physician asked you to stop taking or replaced. Remember to include dosages and the reasons your physician has prescribed them to you. Note any side effects you have experienced. If you think the medications are working (or perhaps are ineffective) make notes so that you can discuss this with your geriatrician.

- Make a list of your concerns and questions. Leave some space for each question so that you can enter your notes during the visit with the doctor in this section.

Bring these documents with you on the day of your appointment. Make sure you pass on the documents to your geriatrician so that he or she can review them with you and store the data in your file. If these documents are the only copies you have, be sure to ask the receptionist to make a photocopy of them and return the originals to you.

During your visit at the geriatrician's office, be patient. You might have to wait a while before you are seen. Sometimes you are called by a medical assistant or nurse into an exam room and asked to wait. You end up sitting in a quiet room with lots of intimidating medical gear and perhaps you start to get nervous. You ask yourself why the doctor is taking so much time to come and see you. You have waited so long for the actual appointment, then waited in the reception area and now continue waiting in the exam room...and you are getting very irritated. Please, do not be alarmed or apprehensive.

My wife was recently seeing a urologist, and during one of her appointments, she was called into the exam room and asked to wait to be seen by the doctor. She waited for a whole hour and nobody showed up! Frustrated, she walked to the receptionist and asked why the doctor was taking so long. She was told the doctor went for lunch! Oops, the nurse said, the doctor forgot to see her! Well, while this happens, it is very rare. The clinicians sitting at the doctor's or nurse's stations are in the process of reviewing other patients' charts (some of whom might have live-threatening problems), ordering tests/referrals/medications, writing notes and discussing patients' conditions with other doctors and health providers. Therefore, be patient. It is unlikely that they have forgotten about you. However, if you have waited for 15 minutes or more and nobody has entered the exam room, feel free to ask the nurse or the medical assistant about the whereabouts of the doctor.

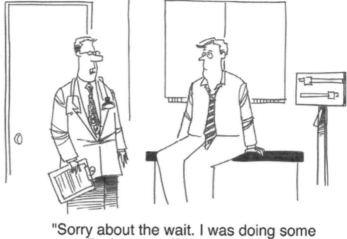

"Sorry about the wait. I was doing some
medical type stuff to another patient."

Once you see the doctor, state the reason for your visit. Don't be shy, scared or embarrassed. Doctors are not gods (not even me, I'm afraid), and therefore, there is no reason to be intimidated. If you feel more comfortable bringing a spouse, friend, or a child with you to the visit, do so. They might be able to bring up issues that skip your mind or even help translate if you do not speak the native language. You can also ask for a professional interpreter if no one is able to accompany you. However, it's not a good idea to bring your *whole* family along since that will just distract both you and the doctor.

Make sure you ask questions if you do not clearly understand any issues discussed by the physician. If the doctor uses medical terminology you do not comprehend, request clarifications. Take notes to make sure you follow instructions thoroughly, and repeat these instructions to your geriatrician to make sure they are correct. You can review these notes later and discuss them with your family members, primary care physician and specialists.

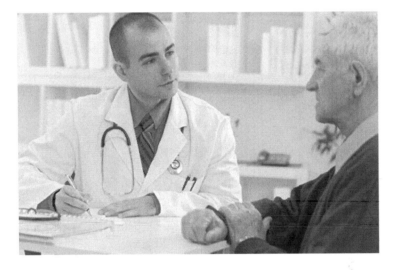

Remember that doctors don't have all the answers or cures. Furthermore, every individual is biologically (in other words, genetically) unique, and therefore, they don't all respond the same to a certain course of treatment or medication. As such, you need to be patient and diligent with your doctor's instructions in order to find what best works for *you* and see the results and benefits. This might take a while. However, if for any reason you do not feel confident about the course of your treatment, try another geriatrician. If you have been patient enough with your doctor and still do not see any positive results or outcomes, or do not feel confident about your geriatrician's knowledge and advice, or do not like his or her bedside manner, or feel intimidated by the physician, *change your doctor*! You need to build a long-term relationship with your physician, and if you dread seeing him or her, and your blood pressure goes up just talking to him or her, then there is no point in torturing yourself! If you believe that your doctor just keeps prescribing medications and tests for you without following up, it is not working out.

I have asked many of my patients about how they go about choosing a physician and whether they are satisfied with him or her once they find one. And the conclusion I have drawn is that there is no scientific way of going about it and there is no guaranteed outcome. You might check a doctor's background, education, publications, accomplishments, experience, and reviews and on paper everything looks great. But once you spend five minutes with him or her, you do not feel confident about his or her medical advice or bedside manner. On the other hand, you might come across a doctor you have never heard of before and just feel she or he is the one. There is no magic formula. We are all unique individuals as are our concerns, expectations and needs. Therefore, what might be a good solution for our closest relatives or friends might not work for us. For instance, I have referred many of my patients to the same specialists and while some are absolutely satisfied with them others are just as unsatisfied. You simply have to try until you find a best fit for you.

That said, I want to leave you with this note. When I was growing up, I remember my father often coming home with fresh eggs, bread baskets, beans, fruits, and vegetables. I once asked why he was going grocery shopping after a long day of surgery and office visits. He proudly smiled and said they were gifts from his patients. I asked him why they were giving him gifts, and he said there were many reasons. A number of his patients were the children or the grandchildren of his previous patients. He had known their families for many years, and they considered him part of their family. The gifts were an act of kindness, trust, and affection. Others could not afford to pay for the visits and instead brought him tokens of appreciation, which he very much cherished and loved. Money is not everything, he would say. Meaningful human relationships are what it is all about.

It goes without saying that you should choose a geriatrician who is well-educated, well-trained, and up-to-date on relevant research and practice. But you need more than that. Have you ever heard of healing hands? My wife swears by this notion. Have you ever gone to see a doctor and just by talking to him or her you felt like a large load had been lifted off your back? You felt ultimate trust and a strong bond. Their kind confident touch, words and caring attitude made a world of difference even when they honestly tell you that they do not have all the answers. That is the type of doctor you are looking for.

ACTION PLAN

1. Prepare a list of questions and concerns you need to discuss with your geriatrician. Leave enough space for each so that you can enter notes during your visit with your geriatrician.

2. Make sure to make notes during your visit with your geriatrician and review them (perhaps with your spouse, family members, or caregiver) when you get home

3. Discuss with your spouse, family members or caregiver whether you feel confident about the care you receive from your geriatrician

This is the first book published from a series of upcoming books by Dr. Ayati and Dr. Azarani. Future publications will cover more topics on the subject of aging including titles such as Aging & Sexuality, Aging & Fitness, and How to Choose the Right Senior Care Facility.

About The Authors

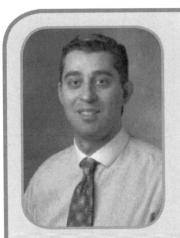 Dr. **M. Ayati** is an Assistant Professor of Medicine at Stanford University School of Medicine. He is Board certified in Family Medicine and Geriatrics. He also practices as a Hospitalist and ER physician at the VA Hospital in Palo Alto, CA. He received his medical degree from the Iran University of Medical Sciences and then came to the US to complete his Internship and Residency program at the University of California, Davis and his Fellowship at Stanford. He is the Medical Director of Los Altos Subacute Care, Sunnyvale Health Center and Palo Alto Rehab Center. His main areas of focus are in improving elderly care and physiology of aging.

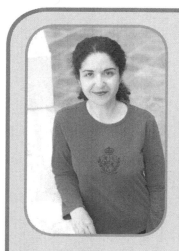

Dr. **A. Azarani** holds a Ph.D. in Physiology from McGill University (Royal Victoria & Shriners Hospital) and Fellowships in Molecular Biology from University of Montreal and Genetics from Stanford University School of Medicine (Department of Pediatric Genetics). She has an Executive Health Care Innovation Management certificate from Stanford School of Professional Development and a Medical Office Manager certificate from Meditec. She has worked for numerous pharmaceutical and biotechnology companies. She has also worked for the Danish Ministry of Foreign Affairs and Ministry of Science and Technology as their Director of Health and Life Sciences in the US.

The two authors, husband and wife, collaborated in creating this book for you. For consistency, the narrator throughout the book is Dr. Ayati, the geriatrician, and when stories of patients appear, they are from his practice. However, the knowledge and experience of both authors are drawn on in the pages that follow.

Made in the USA
San Bernardino, CA
15 March 2015